Homeopathic Medicines for Pregnancy & Childbirth

Homeopathic Medicines for Pregnancy & Childbirth

Richard Moskowitz, M.D.

North Atlantic Books
Berkeley, California

Homeopathic Educational Services
Berkeley, California

ISBN 1-55643-137-6

Published by
North Atlantic Books
P.O. Box 12327
Berkeley, California 94712
and
Homeopathic Educational Services
2124 Kittredge Street
Berkeley, California 94704

Cover photograph © Harriette Hartigan/Artemis
Cover and book design by Paula Morrison
Printed in the United States of America

Homeopathic Medicines for Pregnancy and Childbirth is sponsored by the Society for the Study of Native Arts and Sciences, a nonprofit educational corporation whose goals are to develop an educational and crosscultural perspective linking various scientific, social, and artistic fields; to nurture a holistic view of arts, sciences, humanities, and healing; and to publish and distribute literature on the relationship of mind, body, and nature.

ACKNOWLEDGEMENTS

I dedicate this book to Dorothy Haley, who called me to my first home birth and showed me how it was done; to Laurie Holmes, R.N., C.N.M., a wise healer, great-souled and courageous, who was always there when needed and often gave more than was asked; and to Lauren Fox-O'Neal, R.N., F.N.P., a true and cherished friend, who helped this book get born and carries on its work today.

I would also like to thank Catherine Coulter, M.A., Julian Winston, David Warkentin, P.A., Prof. Barbara Katz Rothman, Judy Norsigian, Linda Cooper, M.D., Peggy O'Mara, and Dana Ullman, M.P.H. for reviewing portions of the text and offering useful criticisms.

Special words of gratitude go to Dana Ullman, whose kindness and sensitivity have been a great solace to me throughout every phase of this long and difficult process.

TABLE OF CONTENTS

PREFACE

The limitations and disadvantages of conventional treatment for many common health problems have prompted more and more people to turn to alternative approaches such as homeopathy. As this book so beautifully demonstrates, homeopathic remedies can be effective in both major and minor ailments during pregnancy, birth, and the postpartum period, and seldom produce the negative side effects and reactions so frequently associated with conventional drugs. Sometimes homeopathy can help prevent problems and complications in ways that conventional cannot match.

As a healing approach that considers how we live, the particular stresses we face, and how we uniquely respond to them, homeopathy also enables and assists us to learn new ways of taking care of ourselves. First with the help of skilled practitioners but in time to a great extent on our own, we can discover for ourselves the remedies most useful for the common problems we encounter.

Recent studies comparing homeopathic remedies with placebo in carefully controlled trials have demonstrated the efficacy of this holistic approach. On the strength of this and other research in the years to come, we expect that homeopathy will attract many more people. Already many women consult a homeopath at the beginning of an ailment or for problems that do not resolve on their own.

Some of our friends have found homeopathy especially effective in dealing with chronic ear infections in small children. Learning how to heal them without repeated use of antibiotics and to reduce the frequency of such infections in the first place has given them a new sense of confidence and competence in caring for their families.

The knowledge and experience we gain from homeopathy not only builds self-confidence but gives a deeper understanding of the healing process. As we debate the subject of a natural health program in the United States and other countries explore the concept of "core services" to be offered as part of a national health system, it is crucial that homeopathy be included on the list of "covered" services. Guaranteeing access to this unique healing approach will improve the health and well-being of many people now unaware of its benefits.

Judy Norsigian and Jane Pincus
Co-authors of *The New Our Bodies, Ourselves*
Spring, 1992

INTRODUCTION

This book grew out of two improbable revivals of the past twenty years. One is the home birth movement, which despite powerful medical opposition has already effected important changes in the sociology and politics of childbirth and women's health in the United States. The other is classical homeopathy, likewise against all odds, which has proved surprisingly popular and versatile as a primary-care vehicle for health professionals and lay people alike. What both movements have in common is a commitment to gentler, more natural models for health care and the healing relationship.

I have used homeopathic remedies since 1974 in more than 800 pregnancies. I have found them to be wonderfully safe and effective in many situations in which conventional drugs and surgery are not required. Yet there exists in English no basic work on homeopathy in pregnancy and childbirth that would be helpful in contemporary home, hospital, or birthing room settings. This is the need that I have tried to satisfy.

I have decided to give primary emphasis to homeopathic self-care of common functional problems that tend to correct themselves spontaneously. In part that is because they are most amenable to the action of natural remedies and therefore least likely to require more drastic methods. They are also the complaints that I have encountered most often in my own experience, which has been limited mostly to home and office settings.

But the most important reason is my conviction that self-healing is the heart of what health care is all about, such that self-care becomes the basic model for client-professional relationships as well. Although at present the book will undoubtedly appeal primarily to a lay audience, I hope and expect that it will eventually be used in hospitals, birth centers, and academic training programs for midwives and childbirth professionals as well.

On the other hand, I have no interest in promoting homeopathy as a panacea for all ills or to the exclusion of other methods. I offer it exactly as I found it —as an elegant and useful technique that deserves to be better known and understood by everyone, lay and professional alike. In particular, it should not be considered an alternative to or substitute for trained and experienced professional help. Yet its tiny and infrequent doses make them more attractive in many situations than pharmaceutical drugs, whose safety in pregnancy and childbirth is usually unknown and must be extrapolated from animal models.[1]

The actual technique of homeopathy involves the use of highly diluted remedies in a manner still not wholly understood. The skepticism and doubt that the method very properly arouses are best answered by the same test that our patients themselves use— namely, does it *work*, does it really help people to heal themselves? I offer this body of experience as evidence that it does. Recent double-blind studies confirm that homeopathic remedies given late in pregnancy tend to shorten labor and prevent dysfunctional patterns and complications more effectively than placebo alone.[2]

The effectiveness of homeopathy in treatment also encourages more humanistic models for thinking about the healing process. Simply including patients' subjective experiences in the definition of health and illness endows their own healing stories with explanatory and indeed mythic power that no mere "placebo effect" can match. For all of these reasons, I will be amply rewarded if pregnant women will simply try homeopathy and see for themselves.

What follows is in no sense a comprehensive textbook of homeopathy in pregnancy and childbirth. The homeopathic *materia medica* already comprises over two thousand remedies, every one a possible candidate for inclusion here. My intention is simply to develop a kit of basic remedies and enough of a methodology to help people get started using them. I have therefore limited myself to those common remedies and conditions with which I have had the broadest personal experience as a solid foundation to build on.

INTRODUCTION

The book is a "primer" in that sense, intended to be used by beginners in homeopathy, both lay and professional, as a basis for further study. I have also tried to develop the remedies in sufficient depth to be useful to homeopaths at all levels of experience. But in neither case should the self-care viewpoint be taken as a substitute for the individualized attention of a trained professional, whether homeopathic or otherwise. The book consists of three sections: 1) a brief introduction to the homeopathic method; 2) a condensed *materia medica* of 25 important remedies, with illustrative cases of each; and 3) an outline of common problems of pregnancy and childbirth with cases and remedies, including some not previously discussed.

Wherever possible, I have tried to illustrate the text with actual vignettes from my own experience, because knowledge of the remedies is built to a great extent on the distinctive features of real people. Looking back on an unforgettable chapter of my life has also been a great pleasure for me and will hopefully serve to bring it to life for others as well.

PART I

Introduction
to Homeopathy

CHAPTER 1

The Law of Similars and Its Implications

Homeopathy is a method of self-healing assisted by small doses of natural remedies and practiced by licensed physicians and other health professionals throughout the world. Homeopathic remedies are protected by federal law and obtainable without prescription for first-aid and domestic use.[1]

The Law of Similars

The homeopathic method was developed by Samuel Hahnemann, M.D. (1755–1843), an eminent German physician and Professor of Pharmacology. In a series of experiments from 1792 onwards, Hahnemann demonstrated

1. that every medicinal substance regularly elicits in healthy people an array of signs and symptoms closely resembling those that it helps to cure in the sick; and

2. that medicines with symptom-pictures most similar to those of a given illness are most likely to initiate a curative response that completes itself spontaneously without further assistance.[2]

Hahnemann understood these experiments to mean that the outward manifestations of illness already represent the concerted attempt of the organism to heal itself, and that the similar remedy acts by reinforcing that attempt in some way. He coined the term "homeopathy" for his method of using remedies with the power to imitate or resonate with the illness as a whole, rather than the conventional method of opposing symptoms with superior force.[3] The Hahnemannian "Law of Similars," *similia similibus curentur*, means "Let likes be cured by likes."

The Law of Similars has never attained general acceptance in medicine, and even those who use it every day accept it as a central mystery not yet explained or proven. Hahnemann himself believed that it would have to be judged by the same empirical standard as all other healing practices, namely, how well it *works* in the treatment of the sick.

In my experience, homeopathy passes this test with the highest honors. Wonderfully safe and effective for a wide variety of common problems, the method also offers a coherent philosophy of health and illness that is accessible to everyone with or without medical training.

Provings

The Law of Similars offers a purely experimental method for investigating the medicinal action of *any* substance, without recourse to either artificial disease models or unconsenting animal subjects. The substance is simply administered to a group of reasonably healthy people in doses sufficient to elicit symptoms without irreversible pathological changes. In this fashion a composite portrait or symptom-picture can be assembled for each substance which is recognizably different from that of every other.

Each homeopathic "remedy" thus represents the composite of all the people who have ever taken it and their detailed responses to it. In this sense it comprises a distinctive "totality" or configuration of health and illness patterns that must be studied as a whole rather than simply as a weapon against a particular disease or group of symptoms.

The Homeopathic Materia Medica

Using himself as well as his family, friends, and colleagues as subjects, Hahnemann compiled detailed and systematic provings of more than ninety medicines in his lifetime, a truly prodigious achievement. The Hahnemannian concept of medicinal action remains the most distinctive contribution of homeopathy to medical science, with important applications to pharmacology and toxicology.[4]

The homeopathic pharmacopoeia presently recognizes more than two thousand remedies, with more being added all the time. A large majority are of plant origin and include flowers, leaves, seeds, roots, barks, and resins. Many are highly poisonous in their crude state, while others are common medicinal herbs, spices used in cooking, fragrances, degradation products (petroleum, charcoal, etc.), mushrooms, lichens, and mosses.

The mineral remedies include metals and other elemental substances, ores, acids, alkalis, salts, and many others (silica, lavas, mineral waters, etc.). The animal remedies include venoms of jellyfish, insects, spiders, molluscs, crustaceans, fish, amphibians, and snakes and other reptiles; secretions, milks, hormones, and glandular and tissue extracts; and disease products or "nosodes" derived from TB, gonorrhea, abscesses, pathogenic bacteria, vaccines, and the like.

The diversity of the homeopathic *materia medica* makes it likely that at least some degree of medicinal help can be found for most people. Moreover, the elegance and simplicity of the investigative method make it equally applicable to the study of folk remedies as yet unproven, as well as conventional drugs, toxic or laboratory chemicals, pollutants, and commercial or industrial products. The *materia medica* is as rich and boundless as the creation of the earth and its transformation and breakdown by human and environmental forces.

On the other hand, although the database of the *materia medica* is enormous, and considerable study is required to practice homeopathy with skill, its basic principles are simple enough that even a novice can obtain creditable results with a small number of remedies. As long as a few commonsense rules and guidelines are observed, the method is perfectly safe for untrained lay people of average intelligence to learn and use at their own pace.

The Totality of Symptoms

The Law of Similars means that an illness cannot be defined in the abstract, apart from the patient who lives through it, and is best understood as a distinctive totality of physical, mental, and emotional symptom-responses, just like the remedies that can help to cure it.

This "totality" need not include every symptom, or any prior assumption about mental symptoms "causing" physical symptoms, or *vice versa*. It is simply a working description of the principal signs and symptoms as they appear, typically mixed up together, and is complete as soon as a reasonable facsimile and a "flavor" or sense of the illness as a whole are discernible.

To the homeopath, this composite totality or psychophysical "style," far more than any abstract disease category or printout of laboratory abnormalities, furnishes the truest picture of the health and illness of the patient, as well as of the particular condition for which treatment is being sought.

The totality of the symptoms means that the choice of a remedy must take into account the lived experience of the patient, the full range of human thoughts and feelings. It by no means rejects or ignores the technical expertise of the physician, and does not hesitate to make use of pathological diagnosis or of conventional drugs or surgery as required. But the technical language of abnormalities is used only to clarify or facilitate the awareness of the patient, not to substitute for it. The patient therefore retains effective control and is encouraged to participate at every step of the process.

The totality of the symptoms also means that the mental and emotional symptoms often weigh heavily in the choice of the remedy. Mental and emotional states designate how human beings feel or function as a whole, such that we say "I am afraid" (or depressed, happy, confused, or whatever) in describing them. Most physical symptoms, on the other hand, refer only to a certain part of the body, so that we speak of "my arm," or nose, heart, throat, "stomach," or back. The totality of symptoms gives special importance to those symptoms which describe the condition of the patient as a whole.[5]

The Single Remedy

The classical or Hahnemannian method employs only one remedy at a time for the whole patient, comparing the totality of symptoms of the patient with those of various remedies until a reasonably
close match is found. The reason is that single remedies can form
meaningful totalities with the richness and individuality of living
patients and are thus most likely to be useful in treatment as well.

Because of its encyclopedic scope, the homeopathic *materia
medica* cannot possibly be learned or grasped in its entirety. In
addition to the various schemes for abbreviating and simplifying
it, there are perfectly competent and reputable homeopaths who
use two, three, or more remedies simultaneously. Compound remedies are also readily available for many simple domestic ailments
and are acceptably safe and effective if properly used.

But the totality of the symptoms is what makes it possible to
accumulate detailed personal experience of the remedies and gen-
erates most of the excitement of learning how to use them. Giving parts of remedies to parts of the patient makes it difficult to
know which remedy has acted, so that remedies have to be selected according to the rough indications of folk medicine or the
technical language of abnormalities, which is not much different
from conventional drug treatment.

Under these circumstances, even when the patient improves,
not much of value will be learned, and what is learned will not add
up to an experience that can build on itself, much less a method
that can be taught. Only the totality of symptoms can display
remedies and patients as unique energy systems supremely wor-
thy of study for their own sake.

The Minimum Dose

Since homeopathic remedies are given less to correct the specific abnormality than to awaken the dormant self-healing mechanism, large or prolonged doses are seldom required and may
actually spoil the effect. Homeopaths use the smallest possible
doses and repeat them only when necessary, allowing the remedies
to complete their action without further interference. Indeed,

the remedy will not work unless it is correctly chosen, unless it fits the illness so closely as to render the patient uniquely susceptible to its action. Otherwise, the minuteness of the dose makes it extremely unlikely that anything untoward or dangerous will occur, an important safety feature.

In a series of painstaking experiments, Hahnemann discovered that remedies continued to be effective at concentrations too small to be measurable chemically, and that mechanical shaking or "succussion" of diluted remedies actually enhanced their healing effect in some way that has never been fully understood. Assuming that the dilute remedies act by stimulating the living organism *qualitatively* on a purely energetic level, he theorized that succussion somehow liberates that energy from chemical "bondage" and releases it into the solution, thus foreshadowing the discovery of subatomic forces in the twentieth century.[6]

Hahnemann's advocacy of "infinitesimal" doses remains one of the most controversial aspects of his work, and many homeopaths have never dared to follow him into this realm. Nor has anyone ever satisfactorily explained how medicines so dilute could possibly have *any* effect, let alone a curative one.

But the standard argument that homeopathic remedies are simply placebos cuts both ways. Quite apart from how they do it, the fact that people regularly heal themselves without drugs or surgery effectively reduces the need for more costly and drastic methods and downsizes the promotional claims made for them. Even now that Hahnemannian microdilutions may be detectable by laser spectroscopy and bioassay,[7] homeopathy still presupposes a new bioenergetic science as yet in its infancy.

The Laws of Cure

The totality of symptoms also explains why drugs that successfully lower the blood pressure, kill bacteria, or do whatever they are supposed to do may still leave the patient feeling as bad or worse than before. Not only our definitions of health and illness but also improvement, worsening, and even the effectiveness of treatment remain essentially ambiguous apart from how patients feel and function according to their own self-imposed standards. Perhaps the greatest failing of modern medicine is its studied unwillingness and inability to address the total energy system of the patient and to follow it through time.[8]

Classical homeopathy studies the totality of the symptoms both anatomically and historically, the order in which symptoms appear, the grouping of symptoms that appear and disappear together, and the relationship of each grouping to the overall health and functioning of the patient.

The formulation most often used today is that of Constantine Hering, M.D., who described four directions in which symptoms often move or redistribute themselves in the process of cure or recovery (falling ill and worsening being opposite):

1. From above downwards, from the head end of the body toward the feet or bottom end.

2. From inside outwards, from more central or interior parts to others more superficial, external, or peripheral.

3. From more vital to less vital organs, from deeper or more important or visceral structures to others less important or indispensable.

4. In the reverse order of their appearance in the life history of the patient, from the most recent to the oldest.[9]

Often confirmed in practice, the first three are successive generalizations of the same basic idea, that healing proceeds by displacing the force of the illness away from the vital centers and toward the less critical areas. The fourth completes them by recapitulating the illness through time, peeling back the layers of illness in the reverse order in which they originally appeared and became chronic or habitual.

Apart from any particular formulation of them, the Laws of Cure are derived from a general assessment of the patient as a whole and thus reaffirm the totality of symptoms over time as the truest and most practical guide for clinician and researcher alike.

CHAPTER 2

Remedies and Patients

Homeopathic Pharmacy

The Homeopathic Pharmacopoeia of the United States (HPUS), 9th Edition, is the official standard for the preparation of homeopathic remedies.[1] Remedies not explicitly conforming to HPUS standards should be regarded with suspicion and reported to the American Association of Homeopathic Pharmacists (AAHP).

Each crude medicinal substance becomes a homeopathic remedy through serial dilution and succussion in a solvent or solid medium. The plant remedies are first crushed or macerated in a specified volume of 95% grain alcohol, then regularly shaken and stored, and the remaining liquid, poured off from the solid residue, is known as the "mother tincture" (abbreviated Ø). The same procedure is used for the animal remedies, nosodes, and any others that are soluble in alcohol.

Substances insoluble in alcohol (e.g., metals, ores) are pulverized or "triturated" with mortar and pestle and diluted with lactose until they become soluble in the manner described below.

The resulting tincture or triturate is then further diluted with alcohol or lactose, according to either of two standard scales. In the *decimal* scale (abbreviated X), a dilution of 1:10 is used, i.e., one part of tincture or triturate to nine parts of alcohol or lactose, and the mixture is shaken vigorously or "succussed" ten times, resulting in the 1X dilution. The same process is then repeated, yielding the 2X, 3X, 4X, and higher dilutions.

The insoluble remedies are triturated in lactose until they become soluble, usually at the 4X to 6X level, and are then dissolved in alcohol for the higher dilutions.

In the *centesimal* scale (abbreviated C), the method of dilution and succussion is exactly the same, but on a scale of 1:100.[2]

In practice, any dilution may be used; but in this country the most popular for self-care are the 6X, 12X, and 30X, representing dilutions of 1:10 6, 12, and 30 times (10^{-6}, 10^{-12}, and 10^{-30}); and the 6C, 12C, and 30C, often written 6, 12, and 30 with the C omitted, representing dilutions of 1:100 6, 12, and 30 times (10^{-12}, 10^{-24}, and 10^{-60}). Most of the higher dilutions for professional work are in the centesimal scale with the C omitted, e.g., the 200th, 1000th, 10,000th, and 50,000th, written 200, 1M, 10M, and 50M, and representing dilutions of 1:100 200, 1000, 10,000, and 50,000 times (10^{-400}, 10^{-2000}, $10^{-20,000}$, $10^{-100,000}$), respectively!

This book emphasizes the lower dilutions primarily (6th, 12th, and 30th), but even the 12C and 30C are already diluted well beyond the Avogadro limit, i.e., out of the ball park of chemistry entirely. Homeopathy in this sense lives on both sides of the boundary between ordinary sense experience and the more elusive, "immaterial" realms of clairvoyance, telepathy, radionics, faith healing, and the like. It is supremely ironic that this most alchemical of therapies was devised by an apothecary and bears throughout the meticulous stamp of that eminently practical profession.

Remedies are typically dispensed on tiny pellets of lactose or sucrose previously impregnated with the alcoholic solution of the substance.[3] They may be taken dry on the tongue, using a moistened fingertip, or dissolved in water and given by the dropperful. The size of the dose and the number of repetitions will be discussed below.

Case-Taking

Time spent with a patient is much more than taking down information or selecting remedies, which may not work or be chosen

properly unless an appropriate relationship and setting are creat-
ed for them. Most people who bear the burden of pain and suffering benefit, first of all, from sharing it with someone who can
understand and appreciate it. Secondly, they often need help to see
a path beyond it, to construct out of what is happening a mythology they can use to guide their healing work. The homeopathic
interview thus can be a powerful healing experience in its own
right, preparing the way for the remedies to continue the process
in the future.

The patient should be invited to tell the story of her illness
in its entirety and allowed to continue without interruption until
she has nothing further to say. The question "What else?" may
be repeated as often as necessary, both to elicit more symptoms
and to remind the patient that no one "disease" but rather the
totality of symptoms is being sought. Symptoms should be written
down, whenever possible in the patient's own words, leaving space
in the right-hand margin for the homeopath's own observations.
The interview follows the outline of the standard medical history and should also include a physical examination and laboratory
work as needed to confirm a pathological diagnosis.

The technique of case-taking is greatly simplified in acute or
first-aid prescribing. Often the past history, family history, and
large sections of the review of systems can be omitted, since the
totality of symptoms need include only what is immediately apparent at the time and what is different in some manner or degree
from the customary pattern. Acute symptoms are also apt to be
fewer in number, more severe or intense, and therefore more readily volunteered by the patient or directly observable through
behavior or body language without having to be elicited by the
interrogation. A half-empty glass, constantly sipped, describes
thirst far better than any verbal report.

Interrogation

When the patient has finished her story and the principal symptoms have been written down, direct questioning may be needed
to characterize them in adequate detail. Questions should be
framed to require thought rather than simple yes-or-no answers.

The interrogation may seem confusing at first, because the conventional pathological diagnosis is based on the common symptoms (fever, pain, cough, bleeding, etc.), whereas the homeopath looks for the odd, unusual, or idiosyncratic features typically overlooked or disregarded for precisely that reason. It is often useful to reassure an anxious patient that she need remember only what she can remember, that her own experience is the object of our search and entirely sufficient to tell us what we need to know.

Fully-characterized symptoms tend to exhibit most or all of the following aspects:

1. Subjective sensations like pain, vertigo, fatigue, or anger often have to be described imaginatively. Pain may suggest an instrument capable of inflicting it, while emotional states can often be illustrated with typical vignettes or behavioral clues such as a friend or loved one might observe. How to help people communicate what they experience is an art that can not really be taught but only shown and practiced.

2. The localization of symptoms (e.g., pains on the same side or alternating sides, that wander, radiate, or are circumscribed and occur always in the same spot) is already well known to most patients, and can often be clarified by studying the body language.

3. "Modalities" are factors by which symptoms are influenced or modified in intensity, e.g., at certain times of the day, from changes in the weather or climate, or from foods, emotional states, or whatever. The abbreviations < and > are used to mean "worse from" and "better from," respectively.

4. "Concomitants" are groupings of symptoms that appear and disappear together, sometimes in a definite sequence (nausea with headache, fever followed by chill, etc.).

Selecting the Remedy

In selecting the remedy, the most important symptoms are usually

a. those which are freely volunteered or exhibited by the patient without careful questioning;

b. those which are most fully characterized and clearly delineated, as above; and

c. those which are most severe or intense and interfere the most significantly with the overall health and functioning of the patient.

Symptoms with these attributes—spontaneity, clarity, and intensity, each indicated by a single underline in the written record—are apt to be of major importance in the illness and therefore in the selection of the remedy as well.

Homeopathic prescribing works by virtue of the seemingly magical correspondence between the database of the medicinal world, the *materia medica*, and the database of the human world, the case record. The genius of the method is that each of these great texts continually illuminates the other. The problem is that there are too many remedies with too many symptoms to be studied or used properly without an encyclopedic memory or a book or computer with the same capacity.

Anyone wanting to access a large number of remedies professionally therefore needs help in proceeding from the clinical totality to the literature of possible remedies to study and choose from. To simplify this task, most experienced prescribers use a "repertory," an index or dictionary of symptoms, each with a listing of the remedies that have elicited it in the provings and/or cured it in practice. By finding the remedies matching the leading symptoms in the case, it is often possible to narrow the search to a much smaller group.

The largest, most comprehensive repertories include all types of symptoms from every anatomical region and physiological system, as well as mental and emotional symptoms (usually the first chapter), "generalities," i.e., physical symptoms or modalities attributable to the patient as a whole (usually the last), and "strange, rare, and peculiar" symptoms (usually mixed in throughout) that often point to the remedy directly.[4]

But the repertory can never be more than a guide to remedies we might not otherwise have considered. Possible remedies must then be studied as a whole, and the final selection should always be based on the evidence of the *materia medica* and the overall or qualitative "fit" of the remedy to the totality of symptoms of the patient, rather than on any purely technical or numerical calculation.

In any case, the acute conditions described in this book do not require detailed repertory analysis, and the *materia medica* presented is concise enough to be accessible without it. Those wishing to study further will eventually need to consult one or more of the standard repertories listed in Appendix I, "Suggestions for Further Reading."

Regimen and Precautions

Dilute remedies are somewhat delicate and sensitive to environmental interference. Although stable in the cold and across a fairly wide temperature range, they can be inactivated by direct sunlight and should be stored in a dark place when not in use, kept dry, and protected from X-rays and other ionizing radiations insofar as possible.

If possible, the mouth should be kept empty of food, drink, toothpaste, mouthwash, tobacco, or any other flavor for at least 30 minutes before and after each dose. Regular or decaffeinated coffee, recreational drugs, and camphorated products (Tiger Balm, Noxzema, etc.) should be avoided throughout the treatment period, even when no remedies are actually being taken. Medicinal herbs may be used occasionally but can interfere if taken daily or on a regular basis. Tea, mild herb teas, alcohol, and tobacco may be used in moderation, as may vitamins and nutritional supplements. Mothballs and other highly aromatic substances (peppermint, menthol, eucalyptus, etc.), strong perfumes, incense, and spices should also be used sparingly.

Conventional drugs often antidote remedies and should be avoided if possible, although an occasional aspirin, antihistamine, or sleeping pill is perfectly OK, and patients requiring maintenance on prescription drugs should not try to discontinue them without medical supervision. Temporary relapse may also follow dental work, especially with drilling and local anesthesia, but in acute conditions the remedy will generally need to be repeated anyway.

Acupuncture and other deep energy therapies may confuse the picture and should probably not be initiated at the same time as homeopathic treatment, but they may be continued for maintenance or added once the effect of the remedies is apparent and can therefore be monitored adequately.

The regimen and mode of life should be kept as simple and healthful as possible, allowing plenty of time for rest, recreation, exercise, and meditation or spiritual practice. Common sense dictates eating and drinking moderately and avoiding highly processed or chemicalized foods and any other substances or circumstances that have been injurious in the past.

Administration and Dosage

Remedies are usually given dry on the tongue in the form of pellets or tablets, or dissolved in water and given by the spoonful or dropperful. The moistened fingertip may be used to extract a small dose (five or ten) of the tiniest granules, resembling candy "sprinkles," which should be allowed to dissolve on or under the tongue. A typical dose of the small pellets would be three or four, and of the medium-sized pellets or slightly larger tablets perhaps two, licked from the palm and dissolved on the tongue. Small children and overly sensitive patients should of course be given less. For a baby, two tablets crushed and dissolved in a cup of water can be given by the spoonful or dropperful as needed throughout the day. But the exact amount or size of the dose is rarely important. Accidental ingestion of even an entire vial is still just one dose and not at all dangerous.

The lower dilutions (6X, 12X, 30X, or 6C, 12C, 30C) are most suitable for acute prescribing in a self-care setting, because they may be repeated as often as necessary and will work to some extent even if only broadly similar to the totality of the case. The higher dilutions should not be repeated as often, must fit the totality of symptoms more exactly, and are more apt to produce "noise" or temporarily disruptive effects. (See below.)

The highest dilutions (10M, 50M) are often known as "high potencies" and the lowest (6X, 12X) as "low potencies," but these terms should probably be avoided, since we cannot know in advance which dilution will be the most potent for a given patient, and receptivity often changes after several repetitions.

In most situations the level of dilution makes little difference. I like the 12C and 30X dilutions for self-care, because they are low enough to be repeated as often as necessary yet high enough to address the subtler forces as well. The higher dilutions are used in chronic cases, where the symptoms are very strong and well-marked or clearly traceable to something that happened long ago. They should not be used in self-care and may be unobtainable without a prescription.

"Dosage" in homeopathy refers mainly to the number of repetitions and has to be tailored to fit the patient just as much as the choice of the remedy itself. The "minimum" dose thus means that we cannot know the correct one until the reaction actually occurs. The general idea is simply to give the remedy until something happens and then stop, allowing it to continue for as long as it can, and repeating it only when the reaction is exhausted.

In acute situations, the remedy should be timed to give the patient a fair chance to respond to three or four doses before changing it, yet repeated soon enough to be able to change it without undue delay, considering the severity of the condition and the rapidity of its evolution.

Thus a high fever of sudden onset in a young infant may call for a remedy every hour or half-hour, and intolerable labor pains or an excruciating headache every 10 or 15 minutes, to allow the usual three or four doses before trying a different one. Conversely, a flu or sore throat developing more slowly over a period of days, or two weeks of persistent nausea and vomiting of pregnancy, may respond better to a four-times-a-day schedule, which allows more time for the reaction to develop. Because we must be guided by the situation, such matters of experience cannot really be taught but are learned and mastered soon enough.

In acute situations such as labor or fever or colic in infants, the remedy often has to be repeated a number of times even after it has acted, since the condition calling for it is likely to continue or to relapse from time to time. It therefore makes sense to taper the remedy as the patient improves and to resume it if she worsens again. If it has not acted after four doses or the picture has changed significantly, another remedy may be chosen, based on the totality of symptoms as before.

Reactions to the Remedy

Often the first indication that a remedy has acted may be some general or nonspecific improvement, such as calming, relaxation of tension, or regaining of strength: the baby with fever drops off to sleep, or the pregnant woman with nausea just feels "more positive," even before the particular symptoms have subsided. Some patients first notice a mild euphoria or feeling of well-being or vitality soon after taking the dose.

Occasionally, one of the presenting symptoms may actually be intensified for a few hours or days, although the patient herself usually feels better and therefore more capable of tolerating it or viewing it with detachment.

In other cases, symptoms may migrate or change according to Hering's Laws of Cure, or snatches of old symptoms may reappear from long ago. But many patients will simply improve without any aggravation and require no further treatment. In all cases, the fundamental criterion for improvement remains the totality of symptoms, including how well the patient feels and functions as a whole, in addition to her specific complaints.

Another common response is simply no response: the condition persists or worsens in the same way as before. Failure to respond after four doses warrants giving another remedy if indicated or re-evaluating the condition and resorting to more drastic methods if necessary. Not infrequently the remedy acts palliatively: the symptoms are relieved somewhat, but the remedy must be repeated often with less and less effect, and the patient otherwise is not much improved. In such cases, the remedy may be changed whenever the patient wishes.

Often the remedy acts well for a time but then "wears off," with the patient relapsing into much the same state as before. If the relapse occurs abruptly or unexpectedly, the remedy may have been antidoted, whether by coffee, drugs, camphor, dental work, a vaccination, toxic chemical, or some emotional or physical stress such as a personal misfortune or exposure to a substance to which she is known to be hypersensitive.

In any case, relapse or return of the original symptoms is the classic indication for repeating the remedy. It signals that the remedy was well chosen and has acted properly. If partial antidoting has occurred, the patient will often recover spontaneously within a few days. Otherwise, the remedy can and should be repeated as before and is very likely to act at least as successfully the second time.

If the first remedy acts well but the illness proceeds into another phase with a different set of symptoms, other remedies will be indicated.

Occasionally the administration of a remedy may be followed by a worsening of the previous symptoms that does not resolve promptly or a general feeling of disharmony or malaise that demands immediate attention. In such cases, a physician should be consulted, and, if necessary, the condition should be stabilized and the patient made more comfortable with whatever conventional drugs are indicated at the time.[5]

Homeopathy: Pros and Cons

There are few if any absolute contraindications to homeopathic treatment. Patients with severe or disabling illness and/or prolonged dependence on conventional drugs are much more difficult to treat even by trained professionals, but such complicated cases need not be considered here. Nor should homeopathy be regarded as a substitute for correction of such structural or mechanical problems as suturing of lacerations, reduction of fractures, emergency surgery, and the like.

On the other hand, homeopathy should at least be considered before resorting to more drastic measures or after conventional methods have failed. In the typical self-care setting, even severe-

ly ill or drug-dependent patients may respond well to acute remedies if they are clearly indicated and their chronic illness or drug
status does not obscure the symptom-picture.

Homeopathic remedies are wonderfully safe, economical, simple to use, and gentle in their action, with notably few serious or
prolonged ill effects. Often subtle at first, the effects of treatment
are nevertheless prompt, thorough, and long-lasting, require infrequent repetition of the dose, and pose minimal risk of chronic
drug dependence. Many patients, friends, and loved ones notice a
general improvement in vitality or well-being and correctly
attribute it to the patient's own efforts, so that recurrence seems
less frightening and indeed less likely.

Nevertheless, homeopathy is far from a panacea for all ills. It is
a difficult and exacting art, and even after years of study and practice a skilled prescriber may need to try several different remedies before obvious benefit is obtained. In other cases, despite the
most conscientious efforts, there is little or no benefit at all. As
already indicated, the remedies themselves are rather delicate
and easily inactivated, so that certain precautions in storage and
handling must be observed.

Finally, and most important of all, we do not understand how the
dilute remedies act, so that it is impossible to predict exactly how a
given patient will respond to a remedy, which symptoms will come
or go, which will change, or in what order. No less than midwifery
or acupuncture, medicine or surgery, homeopathy is above all an
art, having to do with the life energy of individual human beings.

What Patients Can and Cannot Expect

By cultivating the direct personal awareness of the patient, homeopathy empowers and trains the basic instincts of self-care in ways
that more drastic methods seldom permit. The action of dilute
remedies further reminds the patient that healing is always possible
and ultimately determined by unique variables embedded deeply
in the individual, whatever the name or stage of the illness.

On the other hand, people suffering with illness, fear, or pain
can also get "stuck" at any point. With the best of intentions, illness may continue or worsen, and a favorable outcome cannot

be guaranteed by even the most skillful homeopath or any other human agency. In the face of suffering and death or after grievous loss or misfortune, healing may not be possible until we learn to accept what cannot be changed and to remain open to our experience without the judgment of fault or virtue added to it.

The technical problems of using remedies therefore tend to be less difficult and important than "nitty-gritty" human issues that should already be familiar to midwives and parents, like knowing when to ask for help, what to do if the help doesn't make it in time, and how to negotiate those messy or gray areas in which inarticulate assumptions are suddenly put to the test.

Finally, the fact that human beings can respond to dilute remedies means that they can also receive and transmit energy in other ways equally unpredictable and likely to remain so. Self-care makes sense to the extent that both health and illness are lived as processes of self-discovery, that although we cannot know what is going to happen to us in the future, we can trust ourselves to learn whatever we need to know at the time.

PART II

Materia Medica

Homeopathy begins and ends with the study of medicinal substances. With the totality of symptoms, the Laws of Cure, and other basic principles in general use by healers of every stripe, homeopathic philosophy exerts a considerable influence outside the small circle of its adherents. But its method of investigating, preparing, and using remedies remains uniquely its own, speaking a private language both rich and beautiful but accessible only to those taking the trouble to learn it.

While the purpose of studying remedies is to recognize them in the health problems of daily life, the actual method teaches how to distinguish each one from all the others and especially from those most closely resembling it. It therefore proceeds both "horizontally," amassing detailed knowledge of more and more symptoms, and "vertically," organizing them into themes of ever broader and deeper significance. The first task would be quite hopeless were it not being continually rescued by the second; and the latter becomes much easier and more fruitful if certain peculiarities of homeopathic thinking are kept in mind.

First, the Law of Similars is fundamentally dualistic in the sense that every remedy can cause symptoms or cure them, can function as medicine or as poison, depending on the dosage or sensitivity of the patient. Thus remedies helpful for patients who crave certain foods also tend to influence aversion or sensitivity to these same substances. Since remedies encompass certain themes or issues as much as any particular resolution of them, any definition that excludes a particular characteristic or rests smugly on what is already known is likely to mislead or fall short.

Second, our knowledge of remedies is built upon successive analogies between older, more limited formulations of a symptom and its application to other areas of functioning that lead to broadening and eventual redefinition of the symptom itself.

Thus, while usually associated with physical symptoms such as headaches and other pains, the classic BRYONIA modality "worse from movement" is equally descriptive of the typical mental state, which shuns intellectual activity or sensory stimulation of any kind. Indeed it comes to represent the BRYONIA energy pattern as a whole, no matter what the illness, on both sides of the psychosomatic frontier, and thus prior to the mind-body distinction itself. In much the same fashion, the entire *materia medica* is continually growing and evolving to an extent that defies any pat or rigid formulation. Much of the art and fascination of using remedies lies in recognizing the old themes in new and ever more inclusive variations.

Third, simple first-aid remedies may also be useful in chronic states arising from a typical acute episode in the past that failed to resolve. Examples of this "never well since" phenomenon include

1. ARNICA, the classic remedy for blunt trauma to the soft tissues, also used for functional ailments appearing in the wake of such an injury;

2. IGNATIA, the great remedy for acute grief and bereavement, also indispensable in the treatment of many illnesses appearing later as a result of them; and

3. STAPHYSAGRIA, a superb remedy for healing knife wounds, no less beneficial to patients who have never recovered from a surgical procedure in the past.

With almost any remedy potentially useful in this way, the simple perpetuation of acute symptoms over long periods illustrates the importance of "stuckness" as an element in many chronic diseases. Recognizing such patterns also leaves room for self-healing to occur and gives permission to resort to more drastic methods when healing cannot be accomplished otherwise.

Finally, there is no simple rule or formula for calculating which of these possibilities might be most relevant in choosing a remedy for a given patient. Those who have never recovered from physical trauma, grief, or surgery may not benefit from ARNICA, IGNATIA, or STAPHYSAGRIA if their present condition is primarily an intensified version of their pre-existing chronic state and accordingly responds better to the remedy indicated by the totality of symptoms at the time. Because an individual decision must be made in each case, the selection of the remedy is seldom a routine matter.

The remedy pictures in this book are drawn from three sources: the proving literature,[1] clinical cases from my own experience, and toxicological data from accidental or deliberate poisoning or overdose with the crude substance.[2] In principle, any remedy could be useful in the conditions described in this book. Many have been omitted because I have not used them enough in pregnancy or labor to be able to present them adequately. Others having little to do with gynecology *per se* have been included because they come up so often for miscellaneous complaints that I couldn't leave them out.

Each remedy has been presented in outline form, using only a few major themes as a schema for adding more particular symptoms along the way. The faults and limitations inherent in such a selection will hopefully motivate students to consult the standard homeopathic literature and to develop a workable methodology for accessing it. A few more detailed *materia medicas* are listed in the Appendix.

Each remedy in this section should be studied as a whole before trying it for a particular condition. Without matching its unique symptom-totality to that of the patient, the beauty and power of the single remedy will be lost and the selection based on generic or routine indications much less likely to succeed.

CHAPTER 3

Two Childbirth Remedies

While many remedies are useful in the treatment of painful uterine contractions, only two have been shown to produce contractions at regular intervals simulating labor. First introduced into homeopathy from American Indian medicine, both are still used primarily for complaints of or in relation to the great female reproductive cycles of pregnancy, childbirth, and menstruation. With symptoms resembling two basic patterns of dysfunctional labor, they are useful standards against which other possible remedies can be measured and may reasonably be tried when other more specific indications are lacking.

CAULOPHYLLUM
Tincture prepared from the root of *Caulophyllum thalictroides*, N. O. Berberidaceae, blue cohosh or "squaw root."

1. Uterine Dysfunction
The muscle fibers of the mammalian uterus have the unique ability to relax isometrically at their contracted length, such that each contraction further reduces the volume of the organ. Centered in the fundus or upper segment, rhythmic contractions of this type accomplish the splendid athletic feats of normal labor: effacing the lower segment, dilating the cervix, and pushing the

baby into, through, and out of the vagina. After labor, similar contractions expel the placenta and any remaining placental fragments, minimizing further blood loss.

The symptomatology of CAULOPHYLLUM is dominated by abnormal uterine contractions of a familiar and easily recognizable type. While often extremely painful and distressing to the patient, they are centered primarily in the *lower* segment and tend to be sharp or spasmodic in character, brief in duration, and extremely unstable, sometimes flitting about here and there or into the bladder, groins, or thighs. Above all, they fail to dilate the cervix, which remains thick and tightly closed, or to empty the uterus, which relaxes to its former length after each contraction, like any other muscle.

Contractions much like these are commonly seen in prolonged or difficult labors that get "stuck" in the dilatation phase, when the vaginal examination reveals so little objective progress that the attendant is apt to feel embarrassed at having to break the news, and may indeed have been misled by the intense pain and exhaustion or insufficiently attentive to the flabby tone of the upper segment to suspect that the labor was progressing unsatisfactorily.

Case 3.1. After a splendidly healthy first pregnancy, a woman of 24 settled into a slow, desultory labor that never progressed beyond the latent phase. Within minutes of a dose of CAULOPHYLLUM 200 she went into good, active labor and gave birth speedily without further impediment.

2. Muscular Weakness and Trembling

Almost invariably the contractions of CAULOPHYLLUM are associated with signs of generalized weakness or exhaustion, sometimes to the point that the patient can scarcely move or speak, or in any case far out of proportion to any tangible effort or work done. At the same time there is generally some evidence of trembling, shivering, or nervous excitement. In both respects its closest analogue is GELSEMIUM, which often succeeds where CAULOPHYLLUM seems indicated but does not help.

Case 3.2. A woman of 31 completed her first pregnancy and labor without any trouble until the placenta separated, when an hour went by without the slightest contraction or urge to expel it. After six drops of CAULOPHYLLUM Ø, she began to have painful contractions, her right arm shook, and she fell back exhausted into a dreamlike state, but still no placenta. With everyone else out of the room, I spoke to her softly in a soothing voice, and the placenta slid out quietly as the contractions subsided. Thus ended my experiments with CAULOPHYLLUM tincture.

3. Neuralgic and Rheumatic Pains

CAULOPHYLLUM has also relieved neuralgic pains in various locations, mainly in the bladder, vagina, and intestines. Much like the uterine contractions, these are short, sharp or spasmodic, and tend to fly about rapidly from place to place. The remedy also has a rheumatic tendency, with pain, swelling, and stiffness in muscles and particularly the fingers, toes, and smaller joints.

4. Miscellaneous Symptoms

The remedy can produce or relieve weakness of the pelvic muscles or laxness of the suspensory ligaments to the point of actual prolapse. It has also been linked with a profuse, irritating vaginal discharge. All of its symptoms tend to appear more frequently and with greater intensity during pregnancy, labor, and menstruation.

Case 3.3. A woman of 22 had no trouble with her first pregnancy until the 39th week, when she complained of urinary frequency and Braxton-Hicks contractions that awakened her at night and left her with a residual feeling of soreness low in the pelvis. Other symptoms included an itchy discharge with irritation of the vulva and tenderness and swelling of the fingers that made her rings uncomfortable. After a few doses of CAULO-PHYLLUM 30 she easily overcome these difficulties, giving birth a week later with no problems of any kind.

31

CAULOPHYLLUM patients tend to be thirsty, chilly, sensitive to the cold, and markedly intolerant of coffee. While often delicate and nervous with rapid changes of mood, they rarely show emotional symptoms as vivid or distinctive as those of PULSATILLA or IGNATIA. The flavor is more what would be expected in someone exhausted and overwrought from a supreme effort upon which she has staked a great deal and for which she finds herself insufficiently prepared.

5. Therapeutics

CAULOPHYLLUM should always be considered and will often be useful in typical or early cases of uterine dysfunction in which the predominant flavor is one of muscular weakness and nervous exhaustion and there are no more specific indications pointing to other remedies. Although most often thought of during labor, including premature or false labor, this pattern may also appear immediately after the birth, as well as during or after miscarriage or abortion, and in dysmenorrhea or difficult menstruation from the teen years through menopause.

Finally, the remedy corresponds to chronic cases in which nervous excitability and weakness of the female reproductive system promote infertility or repeated miscarriages, premature or dysfunctional labors, or postpartum complications attributable to uterine atony (excessive bleeding, retained placenta, subinvolution, etc.).

For women with a history of this kind, CAULOPHYLLUM 6 or 12 given daily for the last two to four weeks of pregnancy will often facilitate a speedier and more efficient labor. A similar regimen may be used to prevent miscarriage or premature labor if either has occurred in the past or is imminent or threatening.

Because of its documented effectiveness in such situations, some homeopaths advocate giving CAULOPHYLLUM routinely in the last month of pregnancy, especially the first one, when excitement and lack of experience with the labor process could be regarded as additional risk factors. Indeed, many reputable observers claim that such a regimen shortens the average length of labor and reduces the level of discomfort and the risk of significant complications.[3]

Personally, I prefer to avoid using remedies routinely without specific indications over long periods of time. More like a proving than a treatment, these strategies have been known to elicit the same range of symptoms for which the remedies are beneficial. One patient given CAULOPHYLLUM 6 daily for the last month gave birth unattended in the hospital corridor and bled heavily enough afterwards that disciplinary action was considered against the midwife who had prescribed it for her.[4] Such reactions are extremely rare, to be sure, and even the one just cited was easily remedied and could have been avoided if the staff had been properly attentive. Yet the fact that women are entitled to participate in such experiments if they wish only underscores the decisive importance of the birth mythology that each pregnant woman must create for herself in her own way.

If the typical symptom-picture is present, CAULOPHYLLUM may also be effective in the treatment of established uterine dysfunction during or after labor, miscarriage, or menstruation. In such cases the fundus tends to feel relatively flabby even during the contraction, and the usual signs of exhaustion and nervousness are likely to be present. CAULOPHYLLUM 12 or 30 may then be given up to every 15 to 30 minutes until there is definite improvement. But it tends to work best before the condition has progressed too far, when other more distinctive symptoms will often point to another remedy, such as GELSEMIUM.

Given the same general features, CAULOPHYLLUM has proved useful in the treatment of neuralgia, arthritis, and rheumatism of the smaller joints (e.g., fingers and toes), particularly toward the end of pregnancy or after labor, miscarriage, or abortion. It has also been helpful in selected cases of vulvovaginitis with a profuse, irritating discharge, notably in late pregnancy and in young girls before the age of puberty.

It is difficult to present vivid individual cases of this remedy, which tends to be most useful in the lower dilutions either preventively or in typical or early cases before reaching their full development. Just as its mental and emotional features are seldom characteristic and even its well-known physical symptoms are pretty much what would be expected under the circumstances, its action is more apt to be solid and workmanlike than spectacular or memorable. But I would not want to be without it.

CIMICIFUGA

Tincture prepared from the root of *Cimicifuga racemosa* (or *Actaea racemosa*), N. O. Ranunculaceae, black cohosh or black snake root.

1. *Uterine Dysfunction*

Like CAULOPHYLLUM, CIMICIFUGA produces abnormal uterine contractions closely simulating those of dysfunctional labor, and its other symptoms are likewise intensified during and after pregnancy, labor, and menstruation. Just as brief, sharp, spasmodic, painful, and unstable as those of CAULOPHYLLUM, these contractions also dart about from side to side or down into the hips and thighs and are felt most keenly in the lower uterine segment and cervix, which remains rigidly closed and fails to dilate. Finally, it resembles CAULOPHYLLUM in its neuralgias, rheumatic and arthritic pains, trembling, nervous and emotional agitation, and a pervasive and bewildering changeability, with symptoms traveling from here to there or changing into one another or back and forth.

2. *Pessimism, Fear, and Mental Fragmentation*

Yet from its minutest details to their overall "flavor" and style, the fully-developed symptomatology of CIMICIFUGA is so distinctive that it will seldom be mistaken for that of CAULO-PHYLLUM or indeed of any other remedy. This uniqueness is especially evident in two paramount features of the mental and emotional life. By far the commoner and easier to recognize is a sense of moroseness, gloom, or dejection, often manifesting as persistently negative behavior, a pessimistic outlook about everything, or a presentiment of failure or misfortune about the pregnancy, the labor, or the parenting to follow. "I can't do it" or "I can't go through with it" would be a fair verbal rendition, doubtless easily overlooked in the throes of a difficult labor, when such sentiments are rarely absent.

Case 3.4. A woman of 28 was sailing through her first
labor with no problems except for her often-repeated
conviction that she wouldn't be able to finish it. In this
fashion she achieved full dilatation and brought the
baby's head halfway down the vagina before her labor did
in fact come to a complete stop, her prophecy seemingly
fulfilled. With a dose of CIMICIFUGA 30 the birth
followed in a few minutes, as if nothing had happened.

In some cases the dejection feels almost tangible or palpable to
the patient: she may say something like "I feel as if enveloped by
a black cloud" and convey by her gestures and body language that
an actual physical presence is meant. Indeed this kind of somatization or extension of mental states into physical symptoms is
another striking feature of the remedy in all its guises. The "black
cloud" sensation in particular has been repeatedly verified in
headache, depression, and many other circumstances.

But underlying these depressive phenomena often lurk bizarre
and disabling fears that something terrible is going to happen to
her, that she will die or be poisoned by the remedy she is about to
take, or that she will go off the deep end and never be the same
again. Terrifying memories of a previous birth, miscarriage, or
abortion may return to haunt her, or she may reveal little beyond
a tangle of disjointed gestures, speech, and actions that makes
everyone around her fear for her sanity as well. The CIMICIFUGA
state ultimately includes the threat or actuality of a mental breakdown in which the common thread or nexus of experience is frac-
tured into a jumble of random thoughts and feelings, a truly
pitiable state justly to be feared by doctor and patient alike.

Case 3.5. A woman of 29 became pregnant again
soon after a miscarriage. After two episodes of second-
trimester bleeding she grew to term in stable condition
but at 42 weeks was still not in labor. At the prospect of
a hospital birth she was frightened by memories of the
miscarriage and D&C and the premonition that the
greater intensity of labor would push her over the edge
once and for all. When she appeared at my office a few

days later, she was already 6 cm. dilated but wild-eyed and out of control, her speech fragmentary, and her gestures disconnected and woeful. Although remaining clinically psychotic throughout the labor, she made excellent progress on a few doses of CIMICIFUGA 200, gave birth normally, and made a full recovery afterward.

In my experience, alarming or prophetic fear of insanity arising from an unbearably painful or terrifying memory of pregnancy, labor, miscarriage, abortion, or menstruation in the past is a genuine keynote of this remedy, repeatedly verified in practice and often helpful in explaining other symptoms as well. Fear of insanity also cuts so deep as to be well guarded by most patients even from themselves and will seldom be volunteered or elicited readily.

3. Fragmentation and Alternation of Physical Symptoms

A similarly fragmented quality usually underlies the physical symptoms as well. Equally intense in both remedies, the pains and twitches of CAULOPHYLLUM are more finely textured and tend to follow or change into one another more easily, rather like PULSATILLA, while those of CIMICIFUGA are coarser, involving larger "chunks" or fragments of experience that replace one another more abruptly in a jumbled or random fashion. A typical labor pain, for example, might begin well enough, with good focus and intensity, only to vanish before reaching its peak or pass off into a disabling obturator neuralgia or sciatica, or alternate with negative or psychotic behavior. Like IGNATIA, LILIUM TIGRINUM, and PLATINA, CIMICIFUGA is one of the principal remedies for physical symptoms that alternate back and forth with one another or with mental or emotional states.

4. Nervous Excitation and Choreiform Movements

Similarly, while the nervous system is just as hyperexcitable as with CAULOPHYLLUM and as prone to trembling, convulsions, and the like, the involuntary movements of CIMICIFUGA are coarser and jerkier, often involving the basal ganglia and extrapyramidal system (chorea, athetosis, grimacing, etc.). On the physical no less than the mental level, the fragmentation and alternation of large chunks of experience abruptly and at random makes the CIMICIFUGA picture not merely changeable or unstable but positively freaky to the patient herself and to everyone around her. The underlying impression is one of disintegration, of experience coming "unglued" in Humpty-Dumpty fashion, which is apt to cast further doubt about the likelihood of full restitution in the future.

5. Pain: Headache, Neuralgia, Rheumatism, Arthritis

Diverse and often disabling, the headaches of CIMICIFUGA can be centered in the back of the head, extending down the neck, or in the vertex, "as if the top of the head would fly off." No less intense are the neuralgias, typically described as darting or lancinating, "like needles pricking," or "like electric shocks here and there." These too may occur anywhere and change abruptly from one place to another without continuity or warning. Other patients are bothered by numbness or rheumatic-type sensations of bruised soreness, either diffuse or localized in particular bones, muscles, or joints. Many of these symptoms are intensified by movement but also shift to the side or part lain on, making it very difficult for the patient to stay comfortable for any length of time.

6. Miscellaneous Symptoms

In general, CIMICIFUGA patients tend to be chilly, and many of their symptoms are intensified in cold, damp weather, except the headaches, which are more likely to improve in the cold. Typical nervous phenomena (nausea, insomnia, palpitations, numbness, etc.) may be associated. As with CAULOPHYLLUM, uterine complaints are often accompanied by bearing-down sensations with or without actual prolapse and in some cases by excessive bleeding as well.

7. Differential Diagnosis

With its unique combination of uterine dysfunction and physical and mental fragmentation, the fully-developed picture of CIMICIFUGA will rarely be mistaken for that of any other remedy.

Although its uterine and nervous symptoms are technically sim-ilar to those of CAULOPHYLLUM, their freaky and disjointed arrangement or alternation with other symptoms will usually set them apart. While BRYONIA is no less arthritic, PULSATILLA at least as volatile, NATRUM MUR. comparably morose, and ACONITE even more fearful, the "essence" or flavor of CIMI-CIFUGA remains equally distinct from all of these.

Perhaps its closest analogue is IGNATIA, similarly motivated by dejection and fear, with a comparable inventory of headaches, neuralgias, and elusive female symptoms that never quite add up or stay put. But whereas IGNATIA ailments arise from grief and often seem contradictory or impossible, those of CIMICIFUGA are like frightful premonitions of insanity and convey the impres-sion of fragmenting or dissociation. Both stylistically and in its minutest details, there is no other remedy even remotely like it; yet CIMICIFUGA is relatively unknown, seldom thought of, and in less advanced cases easily missed.

8. Therapeutics

CIMICIFUGA should be considered for uterine dysfunction with nervous agitation, neuralgic or rheumatic pains, and the charac-teristic sense of physical and mental fragmentation underlying them. Such a pattern can be seen during prolonged or difficult labor, including premature or false labor; after labor, with typical postpartum complications (bleeding, retained placenta, after-pains, subinvolution); and similarly during or after miscarriage or abortion, menstruation, or menopause.

> Case 3.6. After giving birth to her second child at home, a woman of 28 developed severe, nauseating after-pains which subsided promptly after a few doses of CIMICIFUGA 30. At six months of age the child developed fulminant acute leukemia and died after weeks of admittedly hopeless chemotherapy that nobody had the courage to withhold from her. In her grief the mother told me that she had always felt undeserving of the pregnancy and had often had premonitions that the

child would be taken away. Soon pregnant for the third time, she had another successful home birth but immediately developed a nasty, disabling arthritis of her right wrist that persisted for weeks, had few distinctive modalities to prescribe on, and did not respond to any of the remedies I tried. Although neither of us could find the words to talk about it, I found myself praying that this baby not be snatched from us as well; and after a few doses of CIMICIFUGA 200 her wrist cleared up quickly and easily, as from a minor injury over which too much had been made.

The remedy may also be used preventively where similar complaints have occurred in the past or appear imminent or threatening. In premature labor or threatened miscarriage, CIMICIFUGA 12 or 30 may be given up to four times daily and for days or weeks at a time.

Case 3.7. At 22 weeks in her first pregnancy, an environmentally-sensitive woman of 38 went into premature labor and continued to suffer from frequent, painful contractions despite enforced bed rest and IV terbutaline drips in the hospital. Interspersed with infrequent doses of PULSATILLA, CAULOPHYLLUM, and GELSEMIUM, I gave her mostly CIMICIFUGA 30 once a day for many weeks, nothing elegant or fancy; but she was tickled pink to give birth to a healthy boy at 37 weeks, and so was I.

CIMICIFUGA is also unrivalled in the prevention and treatment of premature labor in women who have borne malformed or defective children in the past. Under these circumstances, CIMICIFUGA 30 or 200 may be repeated weekly as needed at the beginning of pregnancy and also throughout the period of greatest risk.

In acute conditions such as actual miscarriage, difficult labor, or postpartum bleeding, CIMICIFUGA 12 or 30 may be given as needed up to every half-hour or even more often, preferably for at least three or four doses before changing it.

When indicated, CIMICIFUGA is an important remedy for postpartum depression, although by no means the only one, and may be of great benefit even in severe cases requiring psychiatric help. Once again, the total symptom-picture is the most reliable guide. An appropriate professional should be consulted immediately if simple first aid such as CIMICIFUGA 12 or 30 four times daily for a few days is insufficient.

CIMICIFUGA 12 or 30 may also be given when indicated for headaches, neuralgias, and the like, up to hourly for four to six hours, as well as prophylactically after each recurrence.

Finally, CIMICIFUGA must not be overlooked for the treatment of chronic complaints such as headaches, arthritis, neuralgia, depression, infertility, or repeated miscarriage, premature labor, or dysfunctional labor that began in the same way but have continued to develop or have never resolved.

Case 3.8. A woman of 36 developed severe pain in the left ankle following the birth of her daughter by Caesarean section five years earlier. Described as sharp and stabbing, "like a pinched nerve," the pain was connected with her learning of the baby's clubfoot, the mere mention of which still evoked strange grimaces and ominous forebodings she could not or would not identify. More symptoms uncannily reminiscent of her mother's stroke appeared when the latter was hospitalized and subsequently committed suicide. Upbeat and optimistic as long as we avoided these unpleasant subjects, she became unnerved and disjointed whenever I returned to them and seemed to need an exorcism at least as much as remedies. After a brief aggravation, her pains quickly yielded to CIMICIFUGA 10M and 30, as did the fears that predictably rose up in their place. Recently she called to report that she has been in good health ever since and has rarely needed or taken the remedy for over six years.

CHAPTER 4

Two Female Remedies

Widely useful in the complaints of pregnancy and childbirth and of the female reproductive organs in general, PULSATILLA and SEPIA are remedies of universal scope that may be indicated for almost any condition and are often given to men and children as well. Also regarded as "female" because of traditional gender stereotypes, both remedies will need frequent re-evaluation as contemporary psychosexual attitudes continue to evolve.

PULSATILLA
Tincture prepared from the entire fresh and still-flowering plant, *Pulsatilla nigricans*, N. O. Ranunculaceae, the meadow anemone or European windflower.

1. *Easy Changeability*
So named because it sways gracefully in the wind, the windflower corresponds to physical, mental, and emotional symptoms that are excessively changeable and adaptable to any persistent internal or external force. Whatever the symptom, PULSATILLA may be suspected by an almost too-accommodating quality, a tendency to be swayed by the prevailing winds of the moment, whatever their source.

2. Emotional Sincerity

This amenable or agreeable quality is often immediately apparent in the emotional life. Typically affectionate and eager to please, PULSATILLA patients are also easy to like and openly delighted when their good feelings are reciprocated. Unpleasant or painful emotions are no less readily accessible, just as freely expressed, and just as quickly forgotten. Equally capable of bursting into tears from an unkind word and of taking comfort from the warmth of a friend, such a patient could also fight with courage and tenacity if her loved ones were attacked or threatened.

In general, the emotions of PULSATILLA tend to be appropriate to the situation, or at least to approximate what most people would naturally feel under the circumstances. Thus on a happy occasion the PULSATILLA patient might well respond gaily with laughter or tears of joy, while in a moment of sadness the tears would come easily and straight from the heart. Even when frank and open expression of them would be unwise, the true feelings can usually be sensed through the disguise: the outward appearance and behavior faithfully reflect the inner reality.

Indeed, their emotions may be so close to the surface that many patients wish they were better able to control them. Especially during pregnancy or before the menstrual period, PULSATILLA women complain a lot of being "too emotional," too readily unbalanced by their emotions and too vulnerable to stress-related illnesses as a result. This surplus of free emotional energy can make them feel powerless to resist manipulation by others, or uncentered and irresolute in the face of conflicting pressures and desires

> Case 4.1. In the fifth month of her first pregnancy a 23-year-old woman developed a bland, odorless discharge and complained that her vulva and vagina were uncomfortably sore and irritated from sexual activity. Despite having known her lover for only a few months when she became pregnant, she felt sexually alive for the first time and desired physical closeness and affection more than ever before. Far more troubling to her than

the soreness were the out-of-body experiences and fantasies of depersonalization that she had always had at the moment of sexual union. Even at the pinnacle of her happiness, she felt tormented by feelings of helplessness, confusion, awe, and exaltation in the midst of primal forces that she could not understand or control and that readily brought tears to her eyes whenever she spoke of them. Her vaginitis cleared up rapidly after a few doses of PULSATILLA 200, and her fantasies gradually faded and occasioned less guilt as the pregnancy continued. She gave birth normally five months later.

With a built-in tendency to follow the path of least resistance, this emotionally mutable style can also take the form of a flighty instability, a tendency to be carried away by any forceful emotion. PULSATILLA is one of the great remedies for ailments that originate from any emotional stress or upset or from simple emotional *excitement*, such as palpitations from falling in love or insomnia after a heavy date, a birthday party, or a stimulating conversation.

3. Heat, Cold, and Circulatory Instability

Easy changeability in response to internal and external forces is equally characteristic of the physical symptoms. Thus PULSA-TILLA patients tend to feel overheated and "stuffy" in a warm room or in the absence of fresh air; yet they may also be sensitive to the cold, and prone to cold injury (chilblains or frostbite) or vasospasm (Raynaud's syndrome). PULSATILLA feet may be too cold to get into bed without woolen socks, then too hot to remain covered at all, and fidget all night looking for a compromise.

The remedy's affinity for the small arterioles, venules, and capillaries is illustrated by the phenomenon of "mottling" in the skin, areas of increased and decreased capillary circulation co-existing side by side and blending into each other. The confluent rash of fully developed measles is another example. Even commoner are simple flushes of heat (e.g., blushing, "hot flashes") or sudden chills in the body or some part of it. Whether overheated or chilly,

43

PULSATILLA patients tend to be intolerant of warm rooms, to bundle up when cold, and to seek relief in the open air for almost any symptom or complaint.

> *Case 4.2.* Seven months pregnant with her first child, a woman of 29 developed a number of complaints in the heat of the summer. Unusually sweaty and "sticky" all over and listless to the point of inaction on the worst days, she found relief only in a daily swim and frequent cold showers. Other problems included stiffness and soreness in her left hip and sacroiliac at work and in bed at night, obliging her to move or fidget around for relief, and persistent heartburn, especially in the evening after a full meal. Rarely thirsty but somewhat better if she reminded herself to drink, she also noticed herself bursting into tears at the least provocation and wanting more display of affection from her husband than ever before. PULSATILLA 30 was quickly effective in this typical situation, and she sailed through the rest of her pregnancy and gave birth at home with no complications.

4. Restlessness

Another aspect of the volatile PULSATILLA style is an inability to sit or lie still or a habit of continually moving about, sewing, puttering, or doing chores simply to "keep busy." Indeed, whatever their symptoms, PULSATILLA patients tend to be relieved by gentle movement or exercise such as taking a stroll or simply changing position from time to time. Even its numerous arthritic and rheumatic pains, headaches, cramps, and the like often change location or "wander" from place to place rather than being reliably confined to the same area or part.

5. Catarrhal Inflammation

PULSATILLA commonly produces and cures inflammation of the mucous membranes of the eyes, ears, nasopharynx, and respiratory and genitourinary tracts, often with easy and plentiful mucous discharges. These are typically rather thick and yellowish, such as would be seen in a "ripe" cold or a full-blown case of the measles, for which PULSATILLA is very nearly specific. When indicated, it is an excellent remedy for simple colds, URI's, ear infections, and conjunctivitis in babies, children, and adults of both sexes. When the symptoms agree, it is splendid for acute and chronic cystitis and vaginitis as well.

> *Case 4.3.* A six-month-old girl had had a cold for almost a week, with a fever of 104°F., restlessness, and a slight yellow discharge from the right ear. Yet in the midst of her illness she played contentedly, was easily comforted by her mother when in distress, and rewarded me with a big smile when I looked at her. PULSATILLA 30 worked like magic in this typical case.

6. *Indigestion*

The digestion and bowels are easily disordered and prone to symptoms of every description, from nausea, heartburn, indigestion, and gas to abdominal pain, hemorrhoids, constipation, or diarrhea. With a definite preference for small meals and a marked intolerance of overeating, PULSATILLA patients are especially sensitive to rich or heavy foods (meat, fat, gravies, sauces, desserts) but may react badly to milk, bread, fruit, onions, or raw vegetables as well. Frequently thirstless, even with fever, they tend to do better when reminded or encouraged to drink plenty of fluids.

> *Case 4.4.* When her first child died of a cerebral hemorrhage in the first hours of life, a 28-year-old woman became pregnant again within a few months and again developed severe heartburn in her second trimester, especially after a full meal. Tolerably well as long as she was doing something, she noticed that her acidity returned in full force whenever she tried to rest or sleep. As always, she cried easily at the slightest disagreement and had to keep the window open to air out the room and reduce the swelling of her feet. With a number of classic indications for the remedy, she responded beautifully to a few doses of PULSATILLA

200 and completed the pregnancy with no further difficulties, giving birth to a healthy baby this time.

7. Genital, Reproductive, and Hormonal Imbalance

With a special affinity for the genitals and the sexual and reproductive life of both sexes, PULSATILLA is one of the principal remedies for acute and chronic prostatitis, epididymitis, orchitis, and inflammations of the male genitalia in general.

In the female, PULSATILLA affects both the internal and external genitalia (vulva, vagina, uterus, tubes, ovaries, breasts) and the hormonal regulation of the reproductive system as a whole. In veterinary practice it often helps to regulate the estrus or mating cycle if abnormal in either direction. Its affinity for the microcirculation and for changeable emotional states suggests a similar locus of action in humans. When the symptoms agree, PULSATILLA may be useful in almost any disorder of menstruation, menopause, fertility, pregnancy, labor, and nursing.

> Case 4.5. After a successful pregnancy five years earlier, a woman of 27 needed help with irregular menses. Never regular and sometimes absent for months at a time, her cycles had averaged from 35 to 50 days since the birth, with only two in the past eight months despite breast tenderness each month as her time drew near. Also unusually prone to tears, she shed them in profusion while speaking of her hopes for more children. Her only other complaints were mild indigestion from overeating and a series of colds and earaches in bad weather. She had a normal period two weeks after a dose of PULSATILLA 10M and continued to menstruate normally until I lost contact with her a year later

With typical versatility, PULSATILLA symptoms include everything from scanty or missed periods to excessive bleeding, dysmenorrhea, and premenstrual syndrome. Used to dry up the milk when a baby dies or is given up for adoption, it can also help restore the milk when suppressed or deficient following a breast infection. It has saved many pregnancies threatened by first-trimester bleeding, and can also facilitate miscarriage in cases of blighted ovum. Because they can act in either direction, depending on the unique sensitivity of the patient, homeopathic remedies often help a troubled organism clarify which way it is actually going.

With all of its symptoms tending to be at their worst before the period and during pregnancy, PULSATILLA is invaluable in treating a wide variety of complaints at every stage of women's reproductive life. It is one of the truly great and indispensable remedies in homeopathy.

8. *Therapeutics*

When its characteristic indications are present, PULSATILLA is a sovereign remedy for virtually every common complaint of pregnancy. It is excellent for nausea and vomiting, for example, especially when brought on by overeating or rich foods and relieved in the open air.

> *Case 4.6.* Eight weeks pregnant with her third child, a 25-year-old woman was severely nauseated and had to force herself to eat. Especially intolerant of raw vegetables, which would rarely stay down, she felt worse after eating more than a small amount and improved in the cool of the evening. PULSATILLA 30 twice a day was truly miraculous for her: her nausea was gone within a week, her energy revived, and she had no further difficulties.

With the usual indications PULSATILLA is also frequently useful for miscellaneous complaints later in pregnancy, including varicose veins, vaginitis, bleeding, indigestion, and emotional problems, to name only a few.

> *Case 4.7.* In the sixth month of her first pregnancy a 20-year-old woman came to see me for anxiety, shortness of breath, and a tight feeling in her chest that was most intense in the evening and often interfered with sleep. Currently single and living with her parents, who were very supportive, she still received nuisance calls from the

baby's father, imploring her to take him back even though he had left and proved otherwise unreliable. In addition to feeling "silly" and crying for no reason, she kept her windows open all winter, and often had indigestion from overeating or after fried or greasy foods. PULSATILLA 30 was quickly helpful, and by her next visit she was feeling fine. At about 35 weeks she developed a bad head cold and sinusitis with thick drainage that often awakened her in the night to breathe cold fresh air for relief. Once again PULSATILLA 30 saw good service, and she gave birth normally a month later.

When indicated, PULSATILLA is a superb remedy for difficult labor, and without characteristic symptoms to suggest otherwise it is commonly used for incomplete miscarriage or retained placenta with continuing pain and bleeding. In such cases PULSATILLA 30 may be given up to every 15 to 30 minutes as needed.

Almost always prescribed on the basis of the overall symptom-picture, PULSATILLA has such a wide therapeutic range that detailed consideration of its use in particular conditions is best deferred until the following section. At this point I will limit myself to three special applications that the remedy fits closely enough to be tried almost routinely if there are no other symptoms to go on.

First, PULSATILLA will often help to bring on the period when it is late as a result of simple emotional excitement or the fear of being pregnant. A simple regimen such as PULSATILLA 30 four times daily for three days would also support the pregnancy in the event that fertilization has occurred.

Second, it has a well-deserved reputation for turning babies in breech or transverse presentations during pregnancy. If the patient feels well and gives no indications for other remedies, PULSATILLA 30 may be given three times daily for three days, followed by PULSATILLA 200 one week later if necessary.

Case 4.8. A woman of 32 was enjoying a healthy, uncomplicated first pregnancy. At 34 weeks a routine prenatal exam showed the fetus in a breech presentation, which was confirmed by ultra-sound.

Two weeks later, still breech and still completely free of symptoms, she tried PULSATILLA 6 three times daily for four days and experienced tumultuous fetal movements, but the baby did not turn. The following week, PULSATILLA 30 was given on the same schedule with the same result. At 39 weeks, after a round of PULSATILLA 200, she reported no movement at all but awoke on the fourth day with the clear sense that the baby had turned. Less than a week later she gave birth in the normal head-down position with absolutely no trouble.

In such cases the remedy should not be given until 35 or 36 weeks, when the baby would be less likely to turn back again and would probably be viable if the remedy did work. On the other hand, it is much less likely to succeed if given after the presenting part becomes engaged and fixed in the pelvis.

Under these circumstances, PULSATILLA given routinely in the absence of specific indications has been effective around 30 to 40% of the time, and in such cases the labor has generally been smooth and easy and tends to follow within a week or two. Although I am much less sure of this, I also have the sense that babies who remain breech after PULSATILLA or the indicated remedy are somewhat more likely to deliver successfully in that position if allowed to do so.

Finally, PULSATILLA is the first remedy to consider to help dry up the milk and prevent breast engorgement after the birth if the patient is not going to nurse or is unable to continue nursing. It should also come to mind when the milk supply wanes after a breast infection. Given four times daily for up to a week, PULSATILLA 30 or 200 will perform very reliably in either circumstance.

Case 4.9. A 24-year-old woman in her first pregnancy went into labor and gave birth normally, but the baby developed congestive heart failure and died at three hours of life. With the help of PULSATILLA 200 three times daily for four days, her breasts dried up shortly with very little swelling or discomfort. A year later she became pregnant again and had a healthy daughter at home without any complications.

SULPHUR is complementary to PULSATILLA, i.e., closely related and harmonious when given before or after it and therefore often used to complete or extend its action.

SEPIA

Trituration of the ink of *Sepia officinalis*, N. O. Cephalopoda, the cuttlefish.

As with PULSATILLA, all of the symptoms and ailments that call for SEPIA tend to be accentuated during and after pregnancy and before and during the menstrual period.

1. Uterine Prolapse and Bearing-Down Pains

SEPIA regularly produces and cures a sensation of heaviness in the pelvis, a dragging or pulling down that may feel as if the uterus will fall out of the vagina. A more extreme version of this sensation is a regular feature of the second stage of labor, when the impulse to bear down becomes irresistible and the crowning head stretches the muscles of the pelvic floor seemingly beyond their elastic limits. Similar bearing-down pains are described by many women before or during the menstrual period.

SEPIA is also useful in the prevention and treatment of actual prolapse and retroversion of the uterus. Even in the absence of frank malposition, women needing SEPIA frequently complain of a nagging backache or pain with deep penetration when they try to make love.

> Case 4.10. After a miscarriage, three abortions, and a hospital birth, a woman of 32 had her second child at home after a castor oil "induction" and a short labor that was over before I could get there. A month later she complained that whenever she stood up too quickly her uterus felt as if it would fall out of her vagina, and she was forced to sit down and cross her legs for relief. Examination showed marked retroversion and sagging of the uterus but no actual prolapse. She also

complained of a vaginal discharge and of feeling more emotional and tearful from having to care for her husband and two children with no time for herself. SEPIA 200 speedily relieved her discomfort and also helped her renegotiate her needs and duties in a calmer and less helpless frame of mind.

2. Sagging Muscles and Tissues

The SEPIA state often includes analogous indications of other muscles and tissues having lost their proper elasticity and tone. Sagging facial and abdominal muscles, drooping eyelids, pendulous breasts, protruding hemorrhoids, bulging varicose veins, and even various internal organs may feel weighted down or become objectively prolapsed in advanced cases. The general appearance and demeanor readily suggest a person prematurely worn out with caring for others and too little rest or recreation for herself.

A similar quality may be observable in the mental faculties as well. SEPIA patients regularly lament their loss of memory and inability to think clearly or creatively or apply themselves to customary intellectual tasks, as if the mentality itself were sagging or drooping under the weight of wifely or motherly chores.

3. Depression and Irritability

A greenish-black pigment widely used in painting, SEPIA is the inky substance discharged by the cuttlefish to cover its retreat when attacked or alarmed. The emotional style of SEPIA patients similarly tends to be overshadowed by depression, irritability, lack of enthusiasm for favorite activities, and loss of affection for friends and loved ones. Spouses and children are apt to complain that customary duties are performed minimally or without enjoyment, and sexual desire is often minimal or absent at the slightest hint of obligation or expectation. The fundamental impulse is usually to escape by being alone or unencumbered by real or imagined demands of or responsibilities to others.

On the other hand, women needing SEPIA may also feel overly conscientious about family responsibilities and thus genuinely and excessively guilty about any desire or effort to avoid them.

This typical ambivalence helps to explain why SEPIA dissatisfactions are seldom assuaged by words alone.

As volatile as PULSATILLA and as weepy when telling their symptoms, SEPIA patients are much less easily comforted, much more likely to explode in anger instead, and tend to remain disaffected and "turned off" in some way even after the particular outburst is over. More like NATRUM MUR. or IGNATIA in this respect, the general flavor of discontent and depression gives their problems a darker coloration wholly foreign to the more agreeable and light-hearted PULSATILLA style.

> *Case 4.11.* Nine months after the birth of her second child, a 37-year-old woman became pregnant again and had an abortion. Soon after the procedure she developed a loose cough with thick, yellow sputum that made her gag whenever she tried to raise or swallow it. Although wealthy enough to afford live-in help, she disliked the boring routine of parenting the infant and received little help from her husband, a busy consultant who was often out of town. With bitter tears she lamented her disillusionment with marriage and family and with men in general, accurately foreseeing that her husband's indiscriminate flirting would soon lead to trouble. Other objective findings included a retroverted uterus and a large hemorrhoid that protruded after every bowel movement. SEPIA 200, three doses in 24 hours, worked wonders for her: her cough disappeared, the hemorrhoid receded, she started to exercise regularly, and she was able to approach her personal problems in a much more active and energetic frame of mind. When her hemorrhoid came back a year later, the remedy worked even better the second time.

Unless measures are taken to prevent it, the 24-hour-a-day job of caring for a newborn infant in a nuclear family with a spouse and perhaps other children can almost be expected to reproduce some version of the SEPIA state. SEPIA is without peer in the treatment of common postpartum complaints such as backache, hemorrhoids, fatigue, depression, and the like.

4. *Nausea and Indigestion*

With a splendid record in the nausea and vomiting of pregnancy, SEPIA is useful for patients overly sensitive to smells or thoughts of even well-loved foods, and to activity or movement like walking or riding in a car. While often aggravated by overeating and fatty foods especially, the nausea and indeed the SEPIA picture as a whole are regularly brought on or intensified by fasting or skipping a meal and relieved by eating. Ambivalence is thus a prominent feature of the physical symptoms as well.

> *Case 4.12.* A 35-year-old woman became pregnant again soon after weaning her second child, then 22 months old. By six weeks she was exhausted and nauseous before mealtimes and would have to eat a little something to relieve it, but the smell of roast chicken and other favorite foods made her feel even sicker and forced her to lie down and try to sleep. Also sensitive to odors like soap and perfume, she felt better when she remembered to exercise, although at their worst her symptoms immobilized her and made her crabby and apathetic. SEPIA 30 soon wrought an amazing change in her: within two weeks she had regained her strength and appetite, feeling only minor nausea occasionally from strong perfume. She remained in good health and went on to give birth at home without any difficulty.

5. *Need for Physical Exercise*

In addition to eating and quiet time alone, physical exercise is consistently beneficial to most SEPIA patients. Not only sagging muscles and downcast spirits but most other symptoms calling for the remedy will probably be relieved by vigorous physical activity of some kind if the patient is still capable of it. Improvement from exercise is indeed a unifying feature of the SEPIA picture as a whole and should always be looked for in patients for whom the remedy is being seriously considered. Moreover, such light activity as would relieve a PULSATILLA patient will rarely suffice: the SEPIA state is the reverse of mobile and requires something more vigorous than simple motion to reactivate it. If SEPIA patients neglect to run, dance, swim, play ball, or work up a sweat on a regular basis, their general health as well as their particular symptoms will probably suffer for it.

6. Genitourinary Symptoms

All SEPIA symptoms tend to be intensified before the menstrual period, during pregnancy, and after labor. No less than PULSATILLA, SEPIA is an important remedy for PMS and is associated with many female complaints common to both pregnancy and the non-pregnant state, such as vaginitis, cystitis, genital herpes, painful intercourse, and psychosexual problems, when the characteristic symptom-picture is present.

> Case 4.13. A woman of 26 consulted me for irregular periods, the interval averaging 35 to 40 days, often with brownish staining around the midcycle. After a home birth three years ago she had nursed the child for a year, with hemorrhoids and constipation developing and her periods getting off track during that time. Although reluctant to speak about her personal life, she was openly resentful of her husband, who was devoted to the child but highly critical of her and scornful of her opinions, and she could no longer tolerate making love with him. After a round of SEPIA 1M, her periods quickly reverted to normal, while her other symptoms improved significantly, and she herself became much more assertive with her husband. No further treatment was needed.

7. Miscellaneous Symptoms

Patients needing SEPIA tend to be chilly and sensitive to the cold. Despite the wealth of other symptoms SEPIA has produced and cured (colds, allergies, headache, backache, constipation, hemorrhoids, insomnia, etc.), the remedy should not be given unless its distinctive features of stagnation and ambivalence are evident.

8. *Therapeutics*

SEPIA ranks with PULSATILLA as one of the supreme remedies for every phase of pregnancy and childbearing and may be used for almost any particular complaint when its characteristic indications are present.

Unexcelled in the treatment of nausea and vomiting of pregnancy, SEPIA also contains important clues within its symptom-picture that could help explain the phenomenon itself. To accept an embryo that is immunologically foreign and a placenta with hormones that digest the uterine wall as it grows, pregnant women must already learn to subordinate their own personal needs to those of the child, the family, and indeed the species as a whole, an accommodation seldom achieved without some resistance. In that sense, the nausea and vomiting of pregnancy are like the biological prototype of SEPIA's fundamental conflict.

> *Case 4.14.* A devoutly Catholic woman of 22 became pregnant on her honeymoon, almost the first time she made love with her husband. Although birth control and abortion were out of the question, she was by no means eager to have a child so soon. At six weeks she was intensely nauseated by the smell of food and often vomited before breakfast but felt better from eating a cracker or something light. After work she would often feel car-sick on the way home but would not vomit until she felt hungry and smelled the food once again. On SEPIA 30 twice daily she was much better in a week, and when her symptoms returned full force at ten weeks, the remedy acted beautifully once again. She had no further difficulties and went on to give birth successfully at home.

SEPIA may also be helpful for nausea and vomiting later in pregnancy, but severe cases requiring hospitalization and intravenous support will often require other remedies as well. When the same general indications are present, SEPIA is also invaluable for other typical complaints of late pregnancy like varicose veins, hemorrhoids, genital herpes, and vaginitis.

Case 4.15. A 29-year-old woman was 16 weeks pregnant with her fourth child when she consulted me for varicose veins. Although PULSATILLA had been of great help in her last pregnancy, this time it did nothing for her. When doing housework, she could feel her uterus hanging down in the vagina as well as tender bulges in the vulva and right leg, both of which were badly varicosed. A fungus infection on her legs also itched a lot at night. By 20 weeks, after a round of SEPIA 200, the varices were much smaller and less painful, the fungus cleared up, and she had no major complaints. Two months later, she left her husband and was staying with her parents in another town, but she remained well and gave birth at term with no complications.

Case 4.16. A 27-year-old woman in her fifth month consulted me for genital herpes. Since her first outbreak five years ago she had had lesions during periods of stress, but in her first trimester she erupted with several that were painful and lasted longer than ever before. While outwardly happy with her second husband, she had lost all sexual interest after the breakup of her first marriage and shunned every kind of physical intimacy. Recently she had moved into town to finish her studies, while he stayed home to run his business 70 miles away. Aside from playing tennis, running, or swimming, her chief pleasures, she felt best if she remembered to eat regularly. After SEPIA 1M she had the shortest and most painful outbreak of her life, a classic homeopathic aggravation,[1] after which she remained free of lesions and in good health, giving birth normally when her time came. Repeating SEPIA 1M for a small lesion three months later, she had no more in the ensuing two years that she remained under my care.

The underlying issues of stagnation and ambivalence are no less commonly applicable to the needs of the postpartum state, where SEPIA is also without peer in its influence over the whole spectrum of typical complaints, such as subinvolution, fatigue, backache, hemorrhoids, retroversion, cystocele, rectocele, depression, and "burnout."

> *Case 4.17.* A 26-year-old woman had her second child at home without any difficulty, although early in the pregnancy she had suffered from nausea and genital herpes, both of which were relieved by SEPIA 30. At her regular postpartum exam she complained of extreme fatigue and lack of vitality, "as if I had water in my veins," which would improve only when she took time for herself and most of all when she played tennis. SEPIA 200, three doses in 24 hours, worked almost magically in this typical situation.

NATRUM MUR. is complementary. NUX VOMICA is closely related and should be considered for acute complaints arising during the treatment period.

CHAPTER 5

Six Acute Remedies

The remedies in this section are used in many acute care situations such as injuries, fevers, headaches, painful labor, bleeding, and the like. Their special affinity is not so much for pregnancy or women's health as for complaints that appear suddenly and develop rapidly.

ARNICA
Tincture of the fresh plant, *Arnica montana*, N. O. Compositae, leopard's bane.

1. Blunt Trauma: Bruising, Bleeding, and Shock
Used for centuries to promote wound healing, ARNICA produces and cures a syndrome most commonly seen after blunt trauma such as a car accident or a fall from a horse. First, injury to the blood vessels and capillaries produces a feeling of bruised soreness and may result in bleeding, contusions, hematoma formation, and the like. Even when unconscious or stuporous, patients so wounded usually resist being touched or approached too closely.

Second, any powerful impact may blunt emergency reflex mechanisms by which injured blood vessels automatically contract to minimize blood loss, and adrenaline and other hormones are released to mobilize and sustain the organism in its survival mode. Shocked, traumatized patients often seem dazed and unresponsive and can bleed excessively from seemingly minor wounds. ARNICA has no peer in rousing a stunned vital force into potentially lifesaving action and accordingly belongs in every emergency room, ambulance, medicine cabinet, and first aid kit. Although its precise mechanism of action is unclear, its basic principles and indications are easily mastered by any reasonably intelligent ten-year-old.

2. Therapeutics

Its applications to pregnancy and childbirth are numerous and important. ARNICA may be given to the mother after labor for obvious bruising of the labia or vagina, or even preventively after much pushing and straining, a difficult forceps extraction, or simply a big baby and a snug fit, when trauma to the soft tissues seems likely.

> Case 5.1. After a strong and beautiful labor, a 27-year-old woman gave birth to her first child, a boy of nine pounds. ARNICA 30 four times daily for two days effectively minimized soreness, bruising, and discomfort in this common situation.

> Case 5.2. A 25-year-old woman gave birth to her first child after a very short labor with no problems except a jagged laceration that needed extensive repair and much bruising and swelling of the surrounding tissues. ARNICA 30 every four hours helped insure rapid, smooth healing, and within days she recovered from this nasty wound with very little pain or discomfort afterwards.

Under similar circumstances, ARNICA helps to prevent or relieve typical postpartum complications like bleeding, retained placenta, and after-pains, and acts as a tonic for the sore muscles, blunted sensorium, and flattened affect that often follow in the wake of a peak effort. In such cases ARNICA 30 may be given up to every two or three hours or more often for a few days, and as needed after that.

After a difficult or traumatic birth, ARNICA is equally useful for the baby. ARNICA 30 can be repeated every hour or two to reduce a large bruise or cephalhematoma, or as often as every 15 to 30 seconds for respiratory depression, stupor, or unresponsiveness calling for resuscitation.

> Case 5.3. After a desultory first stage, a 24-year-old woman went into active labor within minutes of a dose of CAULOPHYLLUM 1M and gave birth to her first child not long after. The baby, a girl of seven pounds, was moderately depressed with an Apgar of 6, the umbilical cord wrapped tightly around her neck, and a large hematoma of the scalp. Within seconds after a dose of ARNICA 30 she pinked up and began to breathe and move normally; at five minutes her score was a perfect 10; and the hematoma had faded almost entirely by the time I left two hours later.

ARNICA is also splendid for bad falls, concussions, tooth extractions, and before and after major surgery of any kind. Postoperatively it may have to be followed by other remedies such as STAPHYSAGRIA. As a simple protocol for Caesarean section or other major surgery, ARNICA 30 may be given at bedtime the night before and on waking the day of the procedure and repeated as soon as possible afterwards and every two hours for the rest of the day, switching to STAPHYSAGRIA 30 that evening, every 3 to 4 hours as needed for pain in the incision for up to four or five days. Also wonderfully soothing as a lotion, ARNICA tincture may be applied topically to bruised or sore places and rubbed into aching backs (but never in an open wound!).

Finally it should be considered for obscure ailments that originated long ago with an injury or traumatic episode for which ARNICA would have been indicated at the time.

ACONITE

Tincture of the whole plant when beginning to flower, *Aconitum napellus*, N. O. Ranunculaceae, monkshood.

1. *Suddenness and Violence*

In its crude state ACONITE is a powerful heart poison with three distinctive features. The first is the extraordinary rapidity and violence of its action. All of the symptoms and conditions to which ACONITE is homeopathic likewise tend to manifest with suddenness and intensity and to disappear just as dramatically. ACONITE is thus pre-eminently a remedy for acute conditions and indeed for the very beginnings of them, usually in otherwise healthy individuals capable of responding in acute and vigorous fashion.

2. *Fear and Palpitations*

The second great theme of ACONITE is its power to stimulate the heart and arterial circulation into rapid and violent activity, most notably palpitations, tachycardia, and high blood pressure, typically accompanied by panic or terror and a fear of impending death. In most patients needing ACONITE, the heartbeat is rapid and uncomfortably strong, perhaps even palpable through the chest wall; the pulse is hard and bounding; and there is usually some restlessness, apprehension, or fear of death that can itself be dangerous. Conversely, ACONITE is unlikely to help a patient who bears illness calmly or whose heart and pulse are unaffected by it. When indicated, it may also be effective for chronic ailments that originated at the time of a sudden fright or other ACONITE experience in the past.

3. *Fever and Inflammation*

The third characteristic of ACONITE is its association with fever and acute inflammatory states, especially in children. As a primitive response to stress, fever often develops hours or days before mucous discharges appear or micro-organisms can be cultured from them. Most commonly seen in small children after exposure to a cold wind or a hot sun, the classic ACONITE fever may reach 105°F. within a few hours, at which point the heart is pounding and the child sleepless with fear. Other signs of inflammation such as pain, redness, and early localization (tonsillitis, bronchiolitis, croup, or pneumonia) may also be present, but in themselves they would never suffice to indicate the remedy. With exposed skin and mucous membranes typically red and dry, sweating is beneficial but limited to the covered parts, and thirst is variable but sometimes extreme.

> *Case 5.4.* A healthy ten-month-old girl awoke in the night with a fever of 104.8°F. and a croupy cough. Earlier in the day, her parents had taken her for a winter outing but did not anticipate the biting cold wind that came up suddenly. When I saw the child, she was apprehensive, with red face, heart pounding at 140 per minute, breathing rapid and shallow, and cough hard, dry, and resonant, like a foghorn. The lungs were entirely clear. We gave her one dose of ACONITE 30 and never had to repeat it. Within 15 minutes she was sound asleep and did not wake again until morning, by which time the fever was down to 101.6°F. and the heartbeat was 100 and quiet. By afternoon she was afebrile and playing contentedly, showing no sign of ever having been ill.

4. Therapeutics

When indicated, ACONITE is used most often in the treatment of acute febrile illnesses in infants and small children (tonsillitis, bronchiolitis, croup, pneumonia, etc.), when it may be given every 30 minutes or so. It should be considered at the start of any febrile illness that comes on rapidly and with great force, especially soon after a fright or exposure to extremely hot sun or cold wind. Under these circumstances, the indications for ACONITE would include evidence of fear, restlessness, and a rapid, pounding heartbeat.

If these same elements are present, ACONITE may also be useful during labor, if the pains are violent or frightful, or the labor fails to progress as a result of fear or after exposure to a cold wind. After labor, it has been used for violent postpartum bleeding with fear, restlessness, bounding pulse, and gushing or spurting of bright-red blood, and also to rescue acutely depressed infants with opposite indications: pallor, shallow breathing, flaccidity, bradycardia, and stupor. In such cases, ACONITE 30 may be given as often as every 10 to 30 seconds if necessary.

In acute illnesses, HEPAR SULPH. often follows ACONITE and helps to complete its action. SULPHUR is complementary.

BELLADONNA

Tincture of the whole plant when beginning to flower, *Atropa belladonna*, N. O. Solanaceae, the deadly nightshade.

1. Suddenness and Violence

Another of the great vegetable poisons, BELLADONNA acts with as much rapidity and violence as ACONITE, like most illnesses calling for it. Like ACONITE, BELLADONNA is pre-eminently a remedy for acute inflammatory conditions that manifest suddenly and with great force.

2. Brain and Autonomic Nervous System Excitation

Readily distinguished from ACONITE in its focus of action on the brain and autonomic nervous system, BELLADONNA means "beautiful lady" in Italian, the name derived from the medieval beauty secret of using nightshade berries to dilate the pupils and make the eyes appear more lustrous.

In physiologic or toxic doses, belladonna selectively blocks the important parasympathetic nerve ganglia that control the secretion of body fluids and the action of key involuntary muscles. Typical signs and symptoms of belladonna poisoning include blurred vision, dilated pupils, wild-eyed expression, defective swallowing or peristalsis, and excessive dryness of the skin and mucous membranes. Atropine and scopolamine, the chief belladonna alkaloids, are still used preoperatively to dry up mucous membranes and suspend basic vegetative processes.

BELLADONNA may also overstimulate the brain to the point of delirium, mania, or convulsions, with hyperacuity of the special senses (sight, hearing, smell, and taste) and sometimes wild or uncontrolled ideation or behavior. But it seldom elicits terror or the violent heart symptoms so characteristic of ACONITE.

3. Fever and Inflammation

As with ACONITE, most acute ailments calling for BELLADON-
NA are accompanied by fever and the four cardinal signs of inflammation—redness, heat, localized pain, and swelling.

BELLADONNA is also one of the supreme remedies for headache and other pains associated with acute inflammation. Wherever they may be located, the pains of BELLADONNA are typically
bursting, throbbing, or pulsating in nature and exquisitely sensitive
to being bumped or jostled, even by someone sitting down too
close on the bed. Whether an acute boil or infected breast, ear, or
throat, the affected parts usually feel hot and dry and look bright-
red, shiny, and taut with swelling. All essentially congestive, these
BELLADONNA pains and inflammations tend to be aggravated
by heat, especially by exposure to direct sunlight, and by light,
noise, or excessive nervous stimulation of any kind.

> Case 5.5. A woman of 30 had her first baby at home
> without any problems. Six months postpartum she went
> back to work as a bookkeeper but began noticing
> unusual symptoms such as sudden flushes of heat,
> violent stomach ache, and marked sensitivity to bright
> light. One afternoon she developed a blinding headache
> under the lights at a shopping mall, chiefly a pressure in
> the temples and behind the eyes as if her head would
> explode, which was further intensified by bright light,
> noise, or any jarring movement, such as a bumpy car
> ride. BELLADONNA 30 almost instantly relieved the
> headache and her other symptoms as well, and she was
> able to continue working without further interruption.

> Case 5.6. Ten months after giving birth to her second
> child, a woman of 31 developed several large, red, hot,
> tender swellings on both legs following a cold. Within
> 36 hours they had ripened into an angry, multifocal
> cellulitis with a low fever, pulse 120 per minute, and
> shiny, red areas that hurt even when not touched but
> throbbed violently with every step. With the help of

BELLADONNA 30 this dangerous infection vanished in a few hours without a trace.

4. Therapeutics

BELLADONNA should be considered in any acute condition in which the cardinal signs of acute inflammation and central nervous system stimulation are prominent. In difficult labor it is very useful for rigidity of the cervix in athletic women and first pregnancies, with failure to dilate, sensitivity to jar, wild-eyed expression, and other typical BELLADONNA features.

> Case 5.7. In active labor with her second child, a woman of 31 was unable to dilate beyond 7 cm., the cervix remaining quite thick and rigid. Although in superb physical condition and showing no sign of fatigue, she could not tolerate anyone sitting on the bed, which she traversed over and over on all fours, wide-eyed and frenzied, like a wild animal trapped in a cage. One dose of BELLADONNA 30 was enough to help her over this final obstacle, and within 30 minutes she was fully dilated and pushing, the baby following soon after.

After labor or miscarriage BELLADONNA should also be considered for excessive or forceful bleeding, with gushing of hot, bright-red blood. In these conditions, BELLADONNA 30 may be given up to every five or ten minutes, depending on the situation.

In general practice, BELLADONNA is most often used in acute inflammatory conditions with fever, particularly in children (URI, pharyngitis, tonsillitis, "Strep throat") and is almost specific for the prevention and treatment of scarlet fever, which it closely resembles in many details. It is also a superb remedy for acute mastitis in nursing mothers, with high fever and exquisite tenderness of the breast.

> Case 5.8. Although somewhat constipated during the pregnancy, a woman of 22 was quickly relieved by a dose of CALCAREA CARBONICA 200 and had a successful home birth with no problems. About a month later, she

suddenly developed a fever of 103⁰F., with a violent
headache and a hard, painful lump in the right breast,
both exquisitely sensitive to being touched, bumped, or
jostled. Through dilated pupils she reached out to me as
if I were far away. In this situation BELLADONNA 30
every three hours was promptly effective: by morning
her headache and fever were gone, within 24 hours she
was able to nurse comfortably, and she continued to
breastfeed for more than a year without any recurrence.

Case 5.9. After a prolonged second stage for which
CAULOPHYLLUM 1M was very helpful, a woman of 31
had her first baby at home uneventfully. When she
developed mastitis three weeks later, she tried antibiotics
with some success, only asking for remedies when it
recurred in the same place the following week. With two
hard lumps in the left breast and the overlying skin red
and shiny, she could not bear to have them touched or
jostled. A fever of 102⁰F. and a pounding left frontal
headache completed the picture. Within a few hours,
BELLADONNA 30 helped abort this strong and
persistent illness without any recurrence or sequelae.

CALCAREA CARBONICA is complementary.

CHAMOMILLA
Tincture of whole fresh plant, *Matricaria chamomilla*, N. O. Compositae, chamomile.

1. Irritability and Intolerance of Pain
Like ACONITE and BELLADONNA, CHAMOMILLA is useful
primarily for acute inflammatory conditions with or without fever
that present suddenly and violently, especially in infants and small
children. But the violence of CHAMOMILLA is centered primarily in the temperament and almost always manifests as intolerance of pain, whether colic, teething, or earache, when even a
healthy, vigorous, sweet-tempered infant easily turns cross, fretful,
and demanding.

No mere request for food or attention, the CHAMOMILLA cry is a howl of protest that sets teeth on edge and that even the most devoted parenting cannot satisfy. Whether the child arches its back or kicks its feet, flails with its arms, or squirms with the whole body, it may be relieved or even fall asleep when carried about or taken for a ride, only to resume just as vehemently when put down for any length of time.

> *Case 5.10.* A six-week-old baby girl was colicky, fretful, and distended in the evening, when she would nurse frantically, bringing her legs up or arching her back, screamed with pain except when carried in her mother's arms, and would wake up the instant she was put down to sleep. When the mother stopped eating dairy products, the baby improved for a few days but was soon worse than before. CHAMOMILLA 30 as needed was quickly soothing to this child, the mother reporting several nights with no symptoms at all. At eight weeks CHAMOMILLA 200 was given, with even better results. After the mother ate a cheese omelet, the baby had her worst attack ever, but it lasted only two hours, and she never had another. No further treatment was required.

2. Digestive Disturbances

Teething, colic, and other typical CHAMOMILLA complaints often originate in the mouth and digestive system or are accompanied by symptoms of indigestion or disordered bowels, such as gas, rumbling, griping pains, greenish diarrhea, and the like.

> *Case 5.11.* A baby boy of five months was brought in for abdominal pain. Although sleeping well during the day and usually sweet and amiable, he often awoke in the night screaming with pain, spitting up curdled milk, and inconsolable except while being rocked or carried about. This common complaint was quickly remedied by CHAMOMILLA 30 twice daily and did not recur.

> *Case 5.12.* A baby boy of 13 months developed a fever of 103°F. with diarrhea and vomiting that even after five

days had not completely resolved. With new teeth coming in, a situation that had often led to ear infections in the past, the child had many crying spells and screaming fits during which he would arch his back, put his fist in his mouth, and demand to be nursed and carried about for relief. CHAMOMILLA 30 gave swift and sure relief in this case, as in so many others like it.

3. Therapeutics

CHAMOMILLA can be prescribed for almost any acute condition with intolerance of pain and the typical irritability and/or digestive upset. By no means limited to children, it can also work splendidly for women who become cross and irritable during labor, demanding constant help and attention from those at hand yet unable to accept or benefit from them when offered. Such a woman might order her doctor, midwife, husband, or friends out of the room and have to be given a wide berth and allowed to run the show in her own way; but a peace offering of CHAMOMILLA 30 every 15 to 30 minutes doesn't hurt and may help to move things along.

> Case 5.13. After a slow start, a woman of 33 went into active labor with her sixth child. After passing a large quantity of bloody show, her contractions became much stronger, and with each one she screamed abusive epithets at her often wayward husband, who was only too happy to leave the room. With a few doses of CHAMOMILLA 30 to calm her, she speedily got down to business, the birth following in short order and with no trouble.

For infants and small children with teething, colic, earache, or other ailments not requiring professional help, CHAMOMILLA 30 may be given every 30 to 60 minutes, depending on the circumstances, either dry on the tongue or dissolved in a cup of water and given by the dropperful throughout the day. As in any other self-care situation, conditions that persist for days or despite repeated doses of remedies warrant prompt medical attention.

Case 5.14. A baby girl of 15 months was brought in with a fever of 103.2ºF. The illness had begun soon after sitting in the hot sun and getting her finger caught in a door, whereupon she screamed loudly and arched her back, stiffening and falling down unconscious, her eyes rolled back, fists clenched, and lips blue. A few hours later she awoke from a nap pulling at her ears and furious with pain, which was somewhat relieved by being carried about. Examination revealed bilateral otitis media, which quickly resolved with the help of CHAMOMILLA 30 every two hours and did not come back.

GELSEMIUM

Tincture of the root bark, *Gelsemium sempervirens*, N. O. Loganiaceae, yellow jasmine.

1. *Acute Inflammation and Fever: Flu Syndrome*

The range and style of GELSEMIUM are both conveniently epitomized by an ordinary case of "the flu." Compared to those of ACONITE, BELLADONNA, and CHAMOMILLA, GELSEMIUM ailments tend to develop more slowly and typically include fever, chills, achy muscles, sore throat, headache, and other symptoms of upper respiratory infection, gastroenteritis, or both. Above all, there is a prevailing sense of fatigue and muscular exhaustion.

> *Case 5.15.* In her first trimester a 29-year-old woman developed a typical flu syndrome over a period of several days. When I saw her, she was suffering with headache, persistent postnasal drip, sore throat, chills, generalized body and muscle aches, and an extreme lassitude that kept her in bed and virtually unable to walk to the bathroom. In this classic situation, a few doses of GELSEMIUM 200 were enough to help her get back on her feet, and after an otherwise healthy first pregnancy she gave birth at home without any trouble.

2. Muscular Weakness and Nervous Excitement

In its provings, toxicology, and clinical uses alike, GELSEMIUM is usually associated with profound muscular weakness or actual paralysis in some cases. Patients with the sort of flu calling for GELSEMIUM are typically unable to walk or perform their usual duties and tend to relapse frequently when they try to bounce back too soon. The remedy is thus also important in the treatment of chronic fatigue syndrome, particularly when traceable to a flu-like illness in the past.

With a special affinity for the eyes, GELSEMIUM can produce and cure fatigue of both the extrinsic ocular muscles (eyestrain, drooping of the lids) and the autonomic pupillary reflex and muscle of accommodation, in the form of other typical flu symptoms like photophobia, blurred vision, and a glassy expression. GELSEMIUM has also produced and cured paralysis of other muscles both voluntary and involuntary, such as the urinary bladder and respiratory muscles, and has proved invaluable in treating Guillain-Barre syndrome and other neuropathies following certain viral infections or the vaccines derived from them.

The muscular weakness and exhaustion of GELSEMIUM are commonly associated with evidence of simple nervous excitement such as trembling or shivering. Also a leading remedy for ailments resulting from *emotional* excitement, GELSEMIUM corresponds especially to "stage fright" with trembling and chattering of teeth or other signs of nervousness in anticipation of some important opportunity, test, or celebration in the future.

> *Case 5.16.* A 22-year-old woman was seven months pregnant with her first child when she and her husband learned that they would have to vacate their apartment in four weeks. During a thunderstorm a few days later, she developed a migraine-like headache, which began around the left eye and caused her to see blank spots in her visual field but later felt like a cap on top of her head and continued to move around. After she had been in pain for several days, she began to feel as though she were "high" on drugs or had stayed awake all night.

71

GELSEMIUM 30 quickly relieved the headache and did so again when it came back a month later in the course of moving. She nevertheless had the baby right on schedule without any further trouble.

3. Miscellaneous Symptoms

With or without fever, GELSEMIUM patients are typically chilly and thirstless but often feel better from urinating in quantity and should therefore be encouraged to drink their fill. Presumably for its calming effect on their nerves, a stiff drink of whisky, brandy, or alcohol in any form may also be beneficial. Finally, GELSEMIUM has headaches of many descriptions, typically with nervous tension or excitement.

4. Therapeutics

A splendid remedy for dysfunctional labor with failure to dilate, GELSEMIUM will usually be suggested by generalized exhaustion with trembling, shivering, or nervous or emotional excitement in anticipation of all that is still to come. In all these respects, its actions on the female reproductive system resemble CAULO-PHYLLUM in every detail and indeed may be even more striking and easier to recognize. When the clinical picture of generalized fatigue and nervousness is fully developed, or CAULOPHYLLUM seems indicated but fails to act, GELSEMIUM is very likely to be effective. In such cases, GELSEMIUM 30 may be given up to every 15 to 30 minutes as needed.

> *Case 5.17.* In labor with her second child, a woman of 23 had great difficulty overcoming a persistent cervical lip late in the first stage and a posterior presentation that would not turn in the second. GELSEMIUM 30 helped her past both obstacles, and she gave birth quite easily in the end without further complications.

CALENDULA

Tincture of leaves and flowers, *Calendula officinalis*, N. O. Compositae, marigold.

Therapeutics

Like no other remedy, CALENDULA promotes healing of abrasions and lacerations of the skin and mucous membranes, prevents infection, and soothes injured tissues. After labor, a warm aqueous solution of CALENDULA Ø applied locally to open wounds of the vagina and perineum will delight and amaze midwives and patients alike and may be repeated as often as desired. Between soaks, CALENDULA ointment may be used inside episiotomy or wound dressings and changed along with them. Equally indispensable for the care of open wounds elsewhere, including lacerations, abrasions, burns, bedsores, ulcers, and puncture wounds, CALENDULA products deserve an honored place in every medicine cabinet.

CHAPTER 6

Eight Common Remedies

The remedies described in this chapter are important in the treatment of a wide variety of common complaints by no means specialized or limited to women's health. The first six will be considered in pairs and the last two separately.

Two Nervous Remedies:
IGNATIA *and* NUX VOMICA

With a composition of more than 40% strychnine in their crude state, both plants elicit symptomatology dominated by hyperstimulation of the central nervous system, with associated hypersensitivity to alcohol, coffee, tobacco, stimulants, drugs, and chemicals of all kinds. Yet the overall flavor and emotional style of these remedies are poles apart and their respective symptom-totalities so incompatible that they should not be given in succession without interposing some other remedy in between.

IGNATIA

Tincture of seeds, *Ignatia amara*, N. O. Loganiaceae, St. Ignatius' bean.

A native of the Philippine Islands, IGNATIA is indispensable in homeopathy and women's health by virtue of certain underlying themes directly or indirectly traceable to the emotional life.

1. *Grief, Sorrow, and Disappointed Love*

Most patients needing IGNATIA are in the throes of some acute grief, sorrow, or disappointment, and their symptoms are much as would be expected under the circumstances but often exaggerated out of proportion by a romantic, sensitive, or artistic temperament. Whether a friend or loved one has died, left, or proved unworthy, or a cherished dream or ideal become unattainable, the agonizing but unavoidable task of giving up the deepest and most passionate attachments often produces analogously improbable or contradictory manifestations in demeanor and conduct.

Thus the work of grieving may be done in secret, while an exaggerated decorum or reserve is maintained outwardly; or it may betray itself involuntarily or paradoxically at the least appropriate time, by sobbing piteously at some light remark or laughing convulsively in a moment of tragedy or repose. In either case, the result is apt to be still further embarrassment and exaggeration of the same overwrought and contradictory nervous and emotional state that produced the tension in the first place.

> *Case 6.1.* A 48-year-old woman consulted me for acute insomnia and anxiety attacks since the death of her mother one month previously. Two years earlier, with her children on their own, she had divorced her husband of 27 years, moved to another state, and fallen in love with her spiritual teacher. A year later, he broke off the sexual part of their relationship, the most intense and passionate of her life, lest it interfere with their spiritual practices. Although still "very close" for the next six months, he continued to draw further away until their meetings, while still beautiful and precious to her, had become very infrequent. During that time she began to notice pressure and tightness in her chest, neck, and throat, had difficulty sleeping, and had two D&C's for menstrual periods that came every two weeks or failed to come for months at a time. All of these symptoms were acutely intensified after her mother's death, to the point that she resorted to sedatives and

anti-depressant drugs to help her get through the day. Even her impeccably refined and decorous manners could not wholly contain or suppress the passionate sobs of grief that would convulse her body at the most inopportune moments. IGNATIA 1M, three doses in 24 hours, and IGNATIA 30 twice daily as needed, were wonderfully soothing to her: within two weeks she was able to sleep and work without drugs, and within six weeks her recovery was complete.

2. "Impossible" or Contradictory Symptoms

IGNATIA is also a leading remedy for physical and nervous ailments originating from grief, sorrow, or disappointment, when the same themes of contradictoriness and impossibility are discernible in the physical symptoms as well. Thus IGNATIA patients are prone to sore throats that are worse from *not* swallowing, gall bladder attacks relieved by sausages and fatty foods, pain or numbness of a whole hand or foot, and other bizarre or "hysterical" symptoms that defy known anatomic and physiological principles. Other symptoms may alternate back and forth, e.g., with their opposites, or from the physical to the mental level, in similarly odd or inexplicable fashion.

> *Case 6.2.* A girl of ten was brought to see me for a bad sore throat that had been interfering with her sleep for over a week. She reported that she often felt a lump there before lunch and that the sore throat was actually better after eating and hurt most when not swallowing. These incongruities soon led to the further discoveries that her best friend's mother was receiving chemotherapy for breast cancer, that a relative had recently died of breast cancer, and that the girl had recently been troubled with thoughts of illness and death and would often wake in a panic if her mother was not in the room to comfort her. IGNATIA 200, three doses in 24 hours, helped her bounce back from this embryonic illness in a few days. When her symptoms returned a

few months later, she asked for the remedy herself, and this time it acted immediately and did not have to be repeated.

3. Drug Sensitivity, Intolerance, and Abuse

Often extremely sensitive to and intolerant of medicinal drugs and stimulants like alcohol, coffee, and tobacco, IGNATIA patients may instinctively crave them as well. Like NUX VOMICA, the remedy is often indicated for ailments associated with repeated or prolonged use or abuse of drugs or medications in general. When the symptoms agree, it may also be useful in the treatment of allergy or hypersensitivity to trace amounts of environmental pollutants or chemicals endured by most people without obvious difficulty.

4. Miscellaneous Symptoms

Replete with spasms, cramps, twitching, convulsions, nausea, vertigo, headache, neuralgia, insomnia, anxiety, and other "nervous" symptoms, IGNATIA is suitable to individuals who are high-strung by nature and overwrought by circumstances. Loud or repeated sighing is a common and useful keynote. IGNATIA patients are frequently subject to attacks of panic or rage, abrupt or violent mood swings, and (like PULSATILLA and GELSEMIUM) ailments from emotional excitement of any kind. As with SEPIA, they tend to be relieved by physical exercise if they can remember to make time for it. The special senses (sight, hearing, smell, and taste) may be almost unbearably acute.

On the other hand, the remedy can easily be missed because the picture that calls for it so often arises from the suppression of feeling, hides behind a haughty reserve or a beguiling mask of secrecy or denial, and may have to be inferred or suspected from the improbable or contradictory pattern of the symptoms themselves.

5. Therapeutics

IGNATIA ailments are no more or less common during pregnancy than at other times, but the remedy is generally regarded as "female" in somewhat the same sense as PULSATILLA or SEPIA and has important gynecological applications. Prominent among them is amenorrhea, often in the wake of a grief or disappointment. IGNA-TIA is a splendid remedy for the college years and for younger adolescents leaving home for the first time, perhaps for boarding school or a long-awaited summer abroad. Whether the periods become erratic or stop entirely for a time, or mononucleosis or repeated sore throats develop, the young woman takes a leave of absence and goes home to recuperate, only to relapse as soon as she returns to school. The remedy is also unsurpassed for jealousy and spitefulness in young children after the birth of a sibling.

> *Case 6.3.* A 21-year-old college student consulted me for amenorrhea. After developing mononucleosis in the fall of her freshman year, she stopped menstruating until she took a leave of absence and went home in February. Resuming normally all spring and summer, her periods disappeared once more when she returned to school in September and did not come back until after her finals in May. A laparoscopy detected evidence of polycystic ovaries, but she reacted violently to all hormone treatments that were offered. She eventually decided to go back to college and "tough it out" but felt unable to exercise and generally "down" on herself. Already in rebellion against her parents in high school, she had become vegetarian, started a radical coffeehouse, and begun experimenting with drugs, but she remained a gifted student, actually liked college, and earnestly repudiated her own homesickness. Her latest passions were solitary (Zen meditation, reciting poetry to herself), and she not infrequently undercut her own narrative with harsh, discordant laughter at the undeniable absurdity of existence. One dose of IGNATIA 200 was repeated weekly for three weeks, at which point she had her first normal period in three years. She wrote back four years later to say that she had continued to menstruate normally ever since.

IGNATIA is also an important remedy for acute ailments and miscellaneous complaints of pregnancy such as fever, headache, sore throat, or insomnia, often following a quarrel or misunderstanding and with the typical pattern of contradictory symptoms or behavior.

NATRUM MUR. is complementary; NUX VOMICA is incompatible before or after.

NUX VOMICA

Tincture of seeds, *Strychnos nux vomica*, N. O. Loganiaceae, poison nut.

1. *Nervous Hyperstimulation*

Although as rich in strychnine as IGNATIA and no less convulsive and stimulant in its properties, NUX VOMICA is more likely to fit the classic type-A or "macho" personality under the influence of cocaine or amphetamines or simply obsessed with power and mastery. Hyperstimulation of the brain, spinal cord, and peripheral nerves is apt to manifest as muscular tension, edgy and impatient behavior, and measurably increased and accelerated mental activity (thoughts, speech, actions). As with IGNATIA, the senses are often painfully heightened during prolonged bouts of wakefulness, insomnia, or simple restlessness and inability to relax. On the other hand, acute illnesses (colds, "flu," sore throats) or periods of unresponsiveness, fatigue, or "burnout" may also be required to allow the overstimulated, exhausted nervous system to "recharge."

> Case 6.4. A 39-year-old dancer consulted me for recurrent cough and weight loss. When the pressure of performing and traveling made her "frazzled" and unable to sleep or relax, she would stay up late drinking coffee and alcohol and smoking cigarettes and would eventually lose weight or come down with a minor illness that knocked her out for several days and left her painfully constipated thereafter. She said that she always had to be "doing something" and abhorred the idea of simply "wasting time." NUX VOMICA 200, three doses in 24 hours, was almost magically restorative to her in this archetypal situation, although her love of the fast lane necessitated repeating the remedy from time to time.

2. Aggressive, Addictive, and Compulsive Behavior

As if driven by some inner need to surpass themselves, those who need NUX VOMICA tend to be equally unrelenting in work and play and to demand or expect the same speed and efficiency from those around them. Impatient with failure or laxness and often intolerant of moderation or simple human frailties, such people may rise quickly to the top of their corporate or professional hierarchies but exact a heavy toll from themselves and usually from their employees, spouses, and children as well. Rarely content to let things take their course, NUX VOMICA patients often try to impose their compulsive personal drive or professional agenda on anyone in their path and may push them aside without compunction if they cannot or will not follow their instructions to the letter.

Furthermore, the accelerated NUX VOMICA style often requires "uppers" or "downers" to keep it going or tone it down. NUX VOMICA patients are especially apt to be habituated or addicted to coffee, alcohol, tobacco, street drugs, or pharmaceuticals, and also to be sensitive to or intolerant of them and of other chemicals as well. Even more than IGNATIA, NUX VOMICA should be considered for people with serious drug reactions or illnesses resulting from the use or abuse of drugs and medications.

> *Case 6.5.* A 36-year-old woman consulted me for a
> stitching pain in her left side that often awakened her at
> 3 A.M. and reminded her of acute hepatitis 11 years
> earlier, in the course of which she had lapsed into a coma
> and nearly died. Since her husband's business reverses she
> was attempting to support both of them on her meager
> earnings and felt generally angry and stressed as a result.
> Although she had not smoked tobacco for several years,
> she did enjoy marijuana at least twice a week and drank
> several glasses of wine daily. Also on the chilly side, she
> was very sensitive to cold, dry, windy weather and to lack
> of sleep, perhaps her biggest problem at the time. With
> the help of NUX VOMICA 30 twice daily she easily
> overcame this stress-related illness in a few weeks' time.

3. Digestive, Rectal, and Bowel Disturbances

With the autonomic nervous system typically on a "wartime" or emergency footing, digestion, elimination, and other vegetative functions are often problematic. NUX VOMICA patients may have very little appetite or may try to get things moving by over-indulgence in rich, fatty, and spicy foods, often suffering gas pains or indigestion as a result. The remedy is also justly renowned for its power to relieve the familiar type of constipation associated with painful urging of a hard stool against a spastic rectum that won't let go. Spasm of the urinary sphincter may also occur.

> Case 6.6. A one-month-old baby girl was brought in for severe constipation of two weeks' duration. Otherwise healthy, nursing well, and gaining weight, this newborn was seldom able to move her bowels at all and then only with grunting, straining, and passing a lot of gas. Over the past few days her efforts to defecate had caused her to scream with pain and frustration, alternatively kicking out her legs and drawing them up to her body. She also startled easily from any sudden noise or bright light or even from being touched. She had a normal stool within an hour after a dose of NUX VOMICA 30, and continued to move her bowels regularly thereafter, without pain or straining.

4. Miscellaneous Symptoms

On the whole, NUX VOMICA patients tend to be chilly and sensitive to cold, dry weather, wind, and drafts, and to benefit from warmth in any form. As a result of overwork, lack of sleep, inability to relax, or intolerance or abuse of drugs, they may be unusually prone to catch colds, sore throats, and other acute ailments. The mucous membranes of the respiratory tract are also frequently sensitized, and hay fever or asthma may develop from exposure to pollen, dander, chemicals, perfume, tobacco, etc. Headaches, back pain, abdominal cramps, muscular tension, insomnia, and nervousness are equally common. All NUX VOMICA symptoms and ailments may be brought on or aggravated by lack of sleep and relieved by a normal bowel movement.

5. *Therapeutics*

Like IGNATIA, NUX VOMICA is a remedy of broad range and universal scope with no particular affinity for childbearing but commonly indicated for miscellaneous complaints and ailments of pregnant women, such as nausea, headache, indigestion, constipation, hemorrhoids, insomnia, and the like. Also very useful in labor, its classic indication is nervous hyperstimulation, often in the form of ineffectual urging for stool with each contraction, only partially relieved by an enema. It should also be considered for babies with colic or constipation and for dysmenorrhea with the typical symptom-picture.

SEPIA and SULPHUR are complementary; IGNATIA is incompatible.

TWO CONNECTIVE TISSUE REMEDIES: BRYONIA AND RHUS TOX

With a similar affinity for the connective tissues (joints, muscles, tendons, ligaments, and fasciae), both remedies are pre-eminently useful in rheumatic and arthritic complaints. In addition, their opposite modalities of motion and rest delimit a fundamental and practical standard against which other connective tissue remedies can be measured.

BRYONIA

Tincture of root before flowering, *Bryonia alba*, N. O. Cucurbitaceae, white bryony or wild hops.

1. *Tissue Affinities*

While most remedies have selective affinities for certain regions, tissues, or organs, those of BRYONIA are peculiar and distinctive. First, it is a leading remedy for inflammation in the membranous lining of the lungs, heart, or abdominal and pelvic viscera— pleurisy and pleuropneumonia, pericarditis, and peritonitis (appendicitis, PID, postpartum infection, etc.). BRYONIA is unexcelled in the treatment of pleurisy with or without underlying lung involvement and will often be effective in cases lacking more distinctive indications for other remedies.

Second, the remedy has an equally marked affinity for the embry-ologically related joint or synovial membranes, including the mus-cles, tendons, ligaments, bursae, and fasciae that support them. In general practice BRYONIA is one of the greatest of the rheumatic remedies and is used most commonly for the treatment of arthritis, bursitis, tendinitis, and other inflammations of connective tissue.

It also corresponds to inflammation of the glands and mucous membranes of the respiratory tract and may be effective in treating sore throat, cough, and flu syndrome when other more characteristic elements are present. In gynecology, BRYONIA shows a definite affinity for the breasts and ovaries and ranks with BELLADONNA as one of the leading remedies for acute mastitis in nursing mothers.

2. Fever with Acute or Subacute Inflammation

As in mastitis, tonsillitis, or flu, BRYONIA is ordinarily most use-ful for acute inflammations with fever, at least in their early stages. But when BRYONIA is indicated the illness is likely to develop more slowly than with ACONITE or BELLADONNA and may even become subacute and require weeks or months to resolve, as is more typical of illnesses like pleurisy, typhoid, rheumatic fever, appendicitis, peritonitis, or pelvic inflammatory disease (PID).

3. Aggravation from Movement

The *sine qua non* of virtually every illness calling for BRYONIA is the grand modality, worse from the slightest movement, or better from being still. This keynote symptom must be prominent to warrant giving the remedy, and in most cases it will be applic-able to the patient as a whole rather than to a single part or symp-tom alone.

Thus the sharp, stabbing or tearing pains of pleurisy for which BRYONIA is nearly specific are aggravated by motion of the chest muscles in breathing, such that the patient prefers to lie on the painful side to splint them. Arthritic joints needing BRYONIA must similarly be immobilized, infected breasts well supported, and the characteristic "splitting" headaches appeased by sitting or lying perfectly still, not even moving the eyes to read.

Case 6.7. Seven months pregnant with her second child, a woman of 25 came in complaining of intense pleuritic pain at the base of her left ribs. Typically very sharp and radiating through to the back, the pain often brought tears to her eyes when she took a deep breath and woke her when she moved in her sleep. Unable to lie on her right side and somewhat relieved by pressure or rubbing, she was most comfortable lying absolutely still on the painful side. These complaints began with a flu-like illness two weeks earlier, and when I saw her she still had a fever of 99.6°F., felt chilly and achy all over, and was very irritable and thirsty, especially for hot drinks. BRYONIA 30 four times daily was splendidly effective in this typical situation, as it was when her symptoms returned a few weeks before the birth, which likewise went off beautifully. She remained well thereafter.

4. *Irritability and Intolerance of Stimulation*

The typical abhorrence of movement can be equally striking in the mental and emotional sphere. BRYONIA patients usually prefer to be left alone, tend to be grumpy or impatient when spoken to or fussed over, and instinctively resist even the minimal effort of having to think or respond. In severe cases, there may be a mild delirium in which the patient appears dazed and lost, perhaps muttering about going "home" to somewhere long forgotten. Above all, they need and thrive on darkness, quiet, and a minimum of mental or sensory stimulation of any kind.

Case 6.8. A 28-year-old woman came in with a flu-like illness and a fever of 101.6°F. Still nursing her second baby, then 13 months old, she developed a stuffy nose, intense headache, fever and chills over the space of three or four days. Described as an intense throbbing or squeezing, the headache became intolerable from the slightest movement or change of position and was relieved somewhat by keeping still and from the pressure of a snug headband. She was also extremely sensitive to loud noise and bright light and unusually short and snappish with her husband and older child, gruffly barking at them to leave her alone. Although quite thirsty, she ate and drank little on account of nausea and a bitter, sour taste in her mouth. BRYONIA 200 four times daily helped this strong illness to resolve quietly in a day and a half.

5. Miscellaneous Symptoms

BRYONIA patients are generally thirsty and appreciate being well provided with drink, both hot and cold, which they may gulp down by the glassful. Not only the mouth but all the mucous membranes tend to be painfully dry and the appetite poor as a result; the patient wants warm soup and liquid food primarily, and the stools are often parched and scanty. Yet BRYONIA patients also tend to prefer their rooms kept on the cool side and dislike becoming overheated. Many complaints are one-sided, especially favoring the right.

6. Therapeutics

BRYONIA is an important remedy in midwifery, not only for flu, bursitis, or pleurisy in pregnant or nursing women, but most commonly for acute or subacute mastitis, with high fever, exquisite pain on motion, and the typical BRYONIA picture. In such cases, BRYONIA 30 may be given up to every one or two hours until better.

> Case 6.9. Since giving birth to her first child three months earlier, a woman of 30 had already had mastitis four times. Although the antibiotics prescribed by her obstetrician had worked promptly each time, the infection always returned soon afterwards in one breast or the other. When I saw her, she had a fever of 104.6°F. with a hot, red lump in the left breast and was sore and achy all over, especially in her wrists, shoulders, and neck, which she tried not to move at all. As with each previous episode, she had a splitting headache behind her eyes which obliged her to keep very still and made it intolerable for her to read or move her eyes. She was

also chilly and thirsty for water, which she gulped down in large quantities. After a single dose of BRYONIA 30 she fell asleep and never had to take another. By morning her fever was gone, the breast was free of pain, and within 24 hours the illness was over for good.

Case 6.10. A 26-year-old woman had twins at home with no serious problems. Seven months later she had a shaking chill as she got up to nurse, her right breast felt very sore, and for the next few days she ran fevers, felt dizzy and nauseated, ate very little, and was immobilized by a sore back and a nasty headache that felt as if she had a clamp around it. What relief she got was from sitting or lying in bed motionless, the slightest movement resulting in vertigo, headache, or vomiting. When I saw her, there was no fever, but she was very thirsty and spoke very slowly, as if from somewhere far away. BRYONIA 30 every two hours was again effective after a few doses, and she was able to nurse her babies for another six months until weaning.

Backed up by hospitalization and conventional treatment as needed, BRYONIA may also be wonderfully effective in early acute appendicitis without evidence of rupture, and in selected cases of rheumatic fever, pericarditis, postpartum infection, or localized pelvic abscess without generalized peritoneal involvement requiring emergency surgery.

RHUS TOX. is complementary.

RHUS TOX.

Tincture of fresh leaves gathered at sunset just before flowering, *Rhus toxicodendron*, N. O. Anacardiaceae, poison ivy.

1. *Tissue Affinities*

Poison ivy commonly produces the familiar blistering dermatitis on contact with the skin of most people, and the plant is indeed useful homeopathically in treating vesicular and pustular skin disorders like impetigo, cellulitis, erysipelas, shingles, and chicken pox.

Much less well-known outside of homeopathy is the plant's equally marked affinity for inflammatory conditions of the joints, muscles, connective tissues (tendons, ligaments, and fasciae), glands, and mucous membranes, with or without fever and swelling. RHUS TOX. is probably the first remedy to be thought of in ordinary sprains, pulled muscles, and stretched tendons or ligaments, if there are no symptoms to indicate any other.

2. Modalities of Motion and Rest and Changes in Weather and Climate

The ailments calling for RHUS TOX. are dominated by two key modalities, both of which will usually be prominent when the remedy is suitable. The first is a pronounced sensitivity to weather changes, particularly to cold, wet weather or the approach of a storm but also to any sudden change in temperature, humidity, or atmospheric pressure. RHUS TOX. patients often predict bad weather very accurately from intensification of their arthritic or rheumatic symptoms and in some cases of other complaints as well.

RHUS TOX. patients are generally chilly, and most of their symptoms are relieved by warm baths, warm blankets, warm rooms, and warmth in any form. Those with rheumatoid or osteoarthritis of the hands, for example, may be comforted not only by drinking hot tea but also by holding the warm teacup against their fingers.

In contrast to BRYONIA, the second RHUS TOX. modality is the tendency of all symptoms and indeed the general condition of the patient as a whole to worsen when sitting or lying still and when just beginning to move and to improve with continued movement.

Many RHUS TOX. patients accordingly find it difficult to rest or sleep or get comfortable in bed, feel stiff on waking, and may experience sharp pain when they first get up from bed or chair or begin to move the painful joint. Once in motion, they often "limber up" and carry on more effectively for a time, but also tire easily once accustomed to the new position or activity, at which point their symptoms are likely to reappear and force them to stop. Typical RHUS patients are thus easily recognized by their inability to stop wiggling, fidgeting, and changing position, their need for repose seldom more than momentarily satisfied.

Case 6.11. A month after weaning her first child, then 13 months old, a woman of 36 developed a nagging pain inside her left elbow that made it difficult to straighten out her wrist without first twisting the arm back and forth to work it out. Described as a sharp "nerve" pain, it was particularly bad when resting or relaxing, in cold, wet weather before a rain or snowstorm, and the day after vigorous exercise, although hardly at all during the workout. With her right leg also stiff and sore before a rain ever since fracturing it, she seemed to be following the example of her mother and two maternal aunts, already crippled with osteoarthritis of the spine. Extremely sensitive to poison ivy since early childhood, she still erupted violently from brushing it lightly with her bare legs. Habitually cold with icy hands and feet, she loved nothing better than to linger in a hot bath whenever she felt unwell. Within days after RHUS TOX. 200 she was no longer troubled by this complaint that had persisted for six weeks without letup and threatened to become a permanent fixture.

3. Miscellaneous Symptoms

Often described as tearing, pulling, or stretching, the muscle, tendon, and joint pains of RHUS TOX. are likely to recur at more or less regular intervals. Indeed, in the literature the remedy is highly esteemed in the treatment of intermittent fever and other complaints that appear at the same hour each day, every second or third day, or with a definite periodicity of some kind. Perhaps most curiously of all, many RHUS TOX. complaints are heralded or accompanied by an inordinate craving for milk.

4. Therapeutics

While it has no particular affinity for pregnancy or childbirth, RHUS TOX. is helpful in such a wide variety of common injuries and complaints of joints, muscles, and connective tissues that it seemed imperative to include it. In midwifery it is useful chiefly for athletic injuries such as sprains and strains, as well as other incidental complications of pregnancy and nursing such as back-ache, tendinitis, arthritis, leg cramps, and sciatica. In such cases, RHUS TOX. 30 may be given three or four times daily, or more often as needed.

Case 6.12. In the ninth month of her first pregnancy a 35-year-old woman came in complaining of back pain, especially on rising and carrying a five-gallon can of water out to the chickens. In recent weeks, while bending down to pick up the eggs, she had felt a "grab" behind her left ribs that often stopped her from getting up yet felt worse when she tried to sit down, leaving her no alternative but to keep going until she worked through it. Also subject to bursitis of her right shoulder in cold, rainy weather, she felt chilly most of the time and addicted to hot baths. She also recalled being "immune" to poison ivy all her life and even rolling in it as a child to show off to her friends. Since becoming pregnant she had developed a strong craving for milk which was most unusual for her. RHUS TOX. 30 twice daily brought her prompt and thorough relief within a few days and was needed only rarely after that. She gave birth on schedule and continued to do well despite a long, difficult labor and her separation from her husband a few months later.

Case 6.13. A 29-year-old woman was 26 weeks pregnant with twins when she came in complaining of aches and pains and inability to sleep. After a hiking trip in the mountains, she noticed that her abdominal muscles were stiff and sore while lying in bed at night and prevented her from falling or staying asleep. Even more annoying was a restless or "jumpy" feeling in her legs that often awakened her and bothered her a great deal whenever she tried to sit in a chair for any length of time. Noticing some relief from her pregnancy exercises, she felt reasonably well as long as she kept moving and avoided becoming fatigued. Since her pregnancy she had also felt chillier and more sensitive to cold, wet weather than ever before. In a very short time RHUS TOX. 30 gave her significant and lasting relief, and she carried the twins to term without further problems. Electing a hospital birth, she delivered them normally and nursed them for over a year without any recurrence.

When the characteristic picture is present, RHUS TOX. is also an important remedy for skin eruptions and infections of a pustular type such as impetigo, cellulitis, erysipelas, shingles, and chicken pox. Somewhat less effective in treating acute poison ivy, oak, or sumac once it has broken out, it is certainly worth trying preventively when exposure seems likely.

BRYONIA and CALCAREA CARBONICA are complementary.

Two Antispasmodic Remedies: AGNESIA PHOSPHORICA and COLOCYNTHIS

Used most often for pain, especially of a cramping or spasmodic type, these remedies also cover much the same range of conditions, from headaches, neuralgia, and sciatica to dysmenorrhea and abdominal or ovarian pain. It also makes sense to study them together because their two characteristic modalities are identical but opposite in order of importance.

MAGNESIA PHOSPHORICA

Trituration of hydrated magnesium phosphate, $MgHPO_4.7H_2O$.

1. Cramps and Spasms Relieved By Heat and Pressure

Perhaps the greatest of the antispasmodic remedies, MAG. PHOS. covers cramps and pains of a spasmodic character virtually anywhere in the body (head, face, teeth, muscles, nerves, back, abdomen, uterus, ovaries) and not much else. Chiefly neuralgic in origin, the pains may also be shooting or lancinating but only rarely burning.

Wherever they are and whatever they feel like, the pains of MAG. PHOS. are characteristically relieved by heat— a warm room, warm blankets, hot drinks, hot baths, or a heating pad—and aggravated by cold. To a lesser extent, the pains may also be relieved by external pressure. Patients with dysmenorrhea may lie in a fetal position with the knees up, while headache or sciatica patients are likely to grasp or squeeze the painful area or ask to have it massaged.

Often accompanying the pain is a vague "nervousness" with anxiety and trembling, which is also relieved by heat. As might be expected, MAG. PHOS. patients tend to be chilly in general, even more so when they are ill, and intolerant of cold in any form.

> *Case 6.14.* Living alone with her three-year-old son, a woman of 36 injured her back in the course of moving to a larger place and began having frequent backaches and sciatica thereafter. When I saw her about a month later, she walked bent over and complained of a persistent squeezing pain down the back of her left leg, as if her sciatic nerve were being pinched very hard. Two closely related symptoms were a left-to-right pain across her lower abdomen and a feeling of tightness and immobility involving the whole of her lower back. Although slightly better from lying on the painful side or on her back with her knees up, she was substantially relieved by heat in any form, especially a hot bath or hot water bottle. MAG. PHOS. 30 made quick work of this disabling complaint: her pain and tension were greatly relieved after three doses and disappeared for good after a fourth a week later.

2. Therapeutics

Often unjustly neglected as a mere palliative, MAG. PHOS. is one of the great neuralgic remedies and one of the simplest to use. It can calm pain too violent and fear too intense for morphine to reach and thus defuse even emergency situations seemingly destined for hospitalization or surgery.

> *Case 6.15.* For the past year and a half, usually on the first or second day of her period, a woman of 22 had had intermittently sharp pains in her right groin, which she described as inflamed and swollen "like a big ball

squeezing," and made her lose control or burst into tears when it shot down into her thigh. Unable to walk or sleep at such times, she was reduced to lying on her back with her knees up, a hot water bottle over the spot, and plenty of codeine. No cyst was ever found. On MAG. PHOS. 30 every two hours she was able to work during her period and needed no Percodan for the next four months. When her symptoms began to come back, MAG. PHOS. 200, three doses in 24 hours, was given preventively at midcycle, her periods became milder, and the remedy was no longer necessary.

In midwifery, MAG. PHOS. is most commonly prescribed for incidental complaints of pregnancy and the nursing period such as toothache, headache, neuralgia, or sciatica. It is also a leading remedy for dysmenorrhea and "Mittelschmerz," endometriosis, and ovarian pain or neuralgia with or without cyst formation.

Case 6.16. After a normal pregnancy and a stillbirth, a woman of 25 developed severe headaches in the last ten days of her third pregnancy. Accompanied by tunnel vision and sparkles of light in both eyes, they were described as throbbing in the temples and behind the eyes and sometimes as crackling or bubbling in the sinuses. Although she managed to give birth normally, the headaches returned in full force a week later, and she decided to seek treatment. Because her only relief came from hot compresses and having the back of her neck rubbed, MAG. PHOS. 30 was given every two hours and as usual made short work of the problem.

When the typical indications are present, MAG. PHOS. may also be useful in labor and should not be neglected in infantile colic and the "stomach aches" of older children. In such cases, the remedy will usually be thought of for neuralgic or cramping pain with the classic modalities and often of such severity that the patient may cry out. A typical dosage schedule for acute pain might be MAG. PHOS. 30 every 15 to 30 minutes until better.

COLOCYNTHIS

Tincture of fruit pulp, *Cucumis colocynthis*, N.O. Cucurbitaceae, bitter cucumber.

1. Neuralgic Pain Relieved by Hard Pressure and Warmth

Like MAG. PHOS., COLOCYNTHIS is an antispasmodic and neuralgic remedy of the first rank and covers much the same therapeutic range, including headache, facial neuralgia, backache, sciatica, and abdominal, uterine, and ovarian pain. Also typically cramping in nature, its pains may likewise be violent in their intensity and are apt to be relieved somewhat by warmth in any form.

But the pains of COLOCYNTHIS are relieved above all by external pressure and especially by hard pressure. Impervious to gentle stroking or massage, the COLOCYNTHIS headache or sciatica may have to be rubbed or squeezed forcefully, while patients with abdominal or uterine pain will pull their knees up tight against the body or press themselves against the top of a chair back or the edge of a table. Infants with colic often require the firm pressure of a hand against the back while lying prone across the parent's knees. More than that of any other remedy, the symptom-picture of COLOCYNTHIS is organized around this key modality, and the remedy should not be given unless it is equally prominent in the case.

> *Case 6.17.* With a long history of diarrhea and cramping with the flow, a 25-year-old woman reported that her periods had become much more violent in the past six months, often with faintness or vomiting from the pain, which forced her to lie "curled up in a ball" on the floor. A heating pad was also somewhat helpful. Typically occurring in paroxysms every ten minutes or so and lasting for up to a full day, these symptoms were frequently accompanied by a "liquid" feeling in her intestines that reminded her of times she had felt frightened or angry; and she generally felt cold, clammy, and exhausted for another day or two afterwards. Only weeks before these problems began, she discovered that

94

her apartment had been broken into and vandalized, and her feelings of outrage and helplessness grew even stronger when she finished her graduate studies and had to submit to the humiliation of several job interviews with as yet nothing to show for them. On COLOCYNTHIS 30, three doses in 24 hours at midcycle and hourly as needed, her periods soon became milder and more regular than they had ever been and her chronic fatigue and intestinal symptoms also disappeared.

2. Anger and Irritability

Many of the ailments calling for COLOCYNTHIS also have a clearly psychosomatic component. Whether or not the patients themselves are aware of the connection, COLOCYNTHIS illnesses often arise from or begin after experiences of anger or indignation and may include uncharacteristic outbursts of temper or irritability displaced onto others or elaborated into an angry predisposition or attitude.

Case 6.18. After a prolonged second stage for which KALI CARB. and CHAMOMILLA were very helpful, a 20-year-old woman had a successful home birth. Four weeks later she came in complaining of bleeding and cramping pain that reminded her of labor and was severe enough to double her over and make her dizzy when she tried to get up. Only a few days earlier, her husband had seized her roughly and abused her verbally in a way that shocked and intimidated her. Although free of nausea, indigestion, or any bowel irregularity, she also felt distended with gas and unable to release it. With the help of COLOCYNTH. 30 every two hours, her cramps and bleeding quickly subsided, and she held her own with firmness and maturity in these adverse circumstances, which soon ended in divorce.

3. Colitis and Irritable Bowel Syndrome

Also associated with mucous or bloody diarrhea, flat ribbony stools, and X-ray or clinical evidence of spasm, COLOCYNTHIS can be a splendid remedy for all types of inflammatory bowel disease, notably "irritable bowel syndrome," ulcerative colitis, and ileitis or Crohn's disease.

4. *Therapeutics*

Like MAG. PHOS., COLOCYNTH. is a superb remedy for ovarian pains with or without cyst formation and dysmenorrhea or uterine cramps that are relieved by hard pressure.

> *Case 6.19.* With laparoscopic evidence of endometriosis, a woman of 29 came for treatment of excessive bleeding and pelvic pain. Although hormones had twice been given with good effect, her symptoms promptly returned, and she felt very uneasy taking such strong drugs for months at a time. Usually sharp and spasmodic, the pains occurred sporadically as well as during her menses, were wholly concentrated in the area of the right ovary, and made her crouch down, double over, or apply hard pressure to obtain relief, often with a heating pad as well. The periods were dark, "rich," and thick, with big clots, painful uterine cramps, and lower backache for the first six hours or so. After a violent argument with her boyfriend's sister, who had recently moved in with them against her wishes, her neck muscles had gone into spasm and forced her to take muscle relaxants for a month, and sexual intercourse became painful and infrequent. Indeed, in retrospect she dated her whole flareup from that time. COLOCYNTHIS 200, three doses in 24 hours at midcycle, quickly relieved both the pain and the hormonal and emotional imbalance that seemed to give impetus to it.

Frequently used for neuralgias of many types in pregnant and nursing women (e.g., headaches, sciatica, trigeminal neuralgia, etc.) and occasionally during labor as well, COLOCYNTHIS is also splendid for infantile colic and for the stomach aches of older children with a psychosomatic background.

Case 6.20. Already nursing and growing prodigiously, a six-week-old baby boy was very colicky and wakeful even after the mother was careful to eliminate all milk and dairy from her diet. Day or night and almost randomly he would cry out in pain, pull his legs up hard, and quiet down only when put across his mother's knees with firm pressure applied to his back. Within a week on COLOCYNTHIS 30 four times daily as needed, he had "outgrown" his colic and was feeding and sleeping normally.

With colitis, ileitis, and other severe or dangerous conditions, a physician should of course be consulted.

STAPHYSAGRIA is complementary.

STAPHYSAGRIA

Tincture of seeds, *Delphinium staphysagria*, N. O. Ranunculaceae, stavesacre.

1. *Surgical Wounds*

STAPHYSAGRIA helps cleanly incised surgical and knife wounds to heal rapidly with minimal pain or infection and may be used more or less routinely after major or minor surgery of any kind.

Case 6.21. After a classic first labor, a woman of 21 gave birth at home without any problem except a large second-degree laceration which was repaired under local anesthesia. A week later she complained of sharp pains in the wound every time she urinated and periodic cramping in her hip muscles and lower abdomen on the same side that made her wince and cry out. Most exquisitely tender were the stitches themselves, from which the dreaded needle-like sensations radiated out in all directions. A few doses of STAPHYSAGRIA 30 quickly reduced pain and inflammation and allowed the wound to heal normally.

Also useful in the treatment of miscellaneous or unexplained chronic problems arising after a particular surgical procedure,

STAPHYSAGRIA has rescued many patients who have never been quite the same since their hysterectomy, tubal ligation, C-section, or whatever. With complaints that are often intermittent and tend to elude conventional anatomical or physiological diagnosis, such people are regularly stigmatized or dismissed as neurotic and shunted from doctor to doctor. Yet the authenticity of the syndrome is elegantly corroborated by the action of this little plant under such unfavorable circumstances. By showing what there is to be healed, the study of remedies can also reveal how illnesses are made.

> *Case 6.22.* Effectively disabled with chronic ovarian pain, a 41-year-old woman clearly recalled its origin five months earlier in the days following her tubal ligation, when she developed a pelvic infection that required intravenous antibiotics and a prolonged hospital stay. Ever since that illness, indisputably the worst of her life, she had had terrible burning pains in her right groin with each menstrual period, especially on the first day, with repeated bouts of cystitis in between. Even her restrained and dignified manner and well-chosen words could not hide her anger and resentment against the doctor who had performed the surgery and seemingly ruined her health. Radiating down her right leg, the pain was somewhat relieved by heat and pressure and had also begun to occur on the left side and at other times between the periods, often waking her from sleep. She also felt "mutilated" and "traumatized" emotionally by the whole experience. After STAPHYSAGRIA 1M, three doses in 24 hours at midcycle, her next period was the most intense ever, but the pain lasted for only a few hours and was much more localized. In the ensuing months her periods were scarcely painful at all, her cystitis gradually disappeared, and she remained well thereafter.

2. Ailments from Suppressed Anger

STAPHYSAGRIA is also unexcelled for the treatment of various complaints arising from anger or indignation, especially when these feelings have been suppressed or stifled for any reason. Whether insulted, humiliated, or physically or sexually abused by a parent, employer, mentor, lover, or therapist, such patients have often been deterred from speaking out by shame or fear of reprisal or out of emotional dependence on the offender.

As after surgery, the result may be a definite illness or an assortment of nervous or psychosomatic complaints, ranging from trembling, insomnia, headaches, irritability, and abdominal pain to actual colitis, cystitis, or prostatitis, held together only by the history of suppressed rage and ongoing humiliation. Indeed surgery itself has to be regarded as a special case if not a prototype of this even more fundamental problem: traumatized by the wound yet prevented by the anesthesia from responding overtly at the time, even an intact nervous system might well be rendered dysfunctional in ways that can seldom be predicted or calculated in advance.

> *Case 6.23.* After a bad case of cystitis while separating from her husband, a woman of 46 remained prone to bladder irritation when she masturbated or made love but could usually rely on a few doses of STAPHY-SAGRIA 30 to take care of it. COLOCYNTHIS 30 had proved equally useful for the sciatica that bothered her from time to time. When I first saw her, she complained of loose stools that drove her from the dinner table and intense, burning pains deep inside the rectum that reminded her of the enemas and suppositories that her mother had applied with sadistic force whenever she misbehaved. In a voice barely audible she confessed that rectal penetration had in fact become secretly erotic for her and always pre-empted her fantasies during sex or masturbation. STAPHYSAGRIA 10M, three doses in 24 hours, was wonderfully comforting to her in the midst of these critical psychotherapeutic issues, and her rectal pain and irregular bowels gradually subsided.

3. Colitis and Irritable Bowel Syndrome

Like COLOCYNTHIS in its propensity for abdominal pain, foul gas, and diarrhea with or without mucus or blood, STAPHYSAGRIA is also an important remedy in the treatment of irritable bowel syndrome, ulcerative colitis, and ileitis, particularly after major surgery or suppressed anger or humiliation.

4. Inflammation of the Genitourinary Tract

Especially prone to cystitis, prostatitis, and other genitourinary infections, patients needing STAPHYSAGRIA are also more likely to develop such ailments after periods of intense sexual activity or masturbation. The so-called "honeymoon cystitis" is a typical example.

> Case 6.24. Complaining of severe itching, burning, frequency, and painful urination, a 33-year-old woman came in demanding that I give her antibiotics. When I told her that I practiced homeopathy and did not prescribe drugs, she scoffed derisively and agreed to try remedies only because she was too impatient to try to get an appointment elsewhere. Following an angry quarrel and two weeks' separation, she had made love with her husband passionately and often the day before she called and had become symptomatic almost immediately thereafter. Apart from a clear discharge and cramplike ovarian pains that scared her when they came, she was wild with the burning that forced her to urinate every 10 or 15 minutes. Although STAPHY-SAGRIA 30 every two hours helped this illness to disappear as fast as it had come, I would never have known it without making the effort to track her down.

With a solid reputation for curing genital as well as other nonvenereal warts, STAPHYSAGRIA is also suitable for some patients who create highly idealized or compelling sexual fantasies that detract from their enjoyment with a live partner.

5. Therapeutics

Used semi-routinely after surgery, including Caesarean section and repair of episiotomies or lacerations of the second degree or higher, STAPHYSAGRIA 30 may be given up to every one to two hours as needed for pain, beginning with ARNICA 30 for several doses before and after major procedures. For cystitis following intense sexual activity or at the beginning of a new relationship, STAPHY-SAGRIA 30 may be given every two to three hours as needed.

Perhaps its most frequent and important application is in the treatment of miscellaneous and often undiagnosed ailments from suppressed anger, for which no universally valid rule or formula need or can be given.

COLOCYNTHIS is complementary.

CARBO VEGETABILIS

Trituration of wood charcoal, C, carbon.

1. Deoxygenation, Decay, and Putrefaction

A residue of combustion, wood charcoal is chiefly elemental carbon in a reduced or deoxygenated state and inorganic mineral ash. As a medicinal agent CARBO VEG. likewise corresponds to pathological states of defective oxygenation in the blood and eventual decomposition and putrefaction in the tissues.

In emphysema, chronic lung disease, or any condition of respiratory failure with inadequate oxygen absorption or transport by the lungs, deoxygenation manifests clinically as marked air hunger and bluish discoloration of the skin and mucous membranes.

> Case 6.25. After a short labor, a woman of 32 gave birth to her second child without any problems, but despite vigorous attempts to breathe the baby remained intensely cyanotic and almost purple in color. Within seconds, my nurse felt sick and vomited, I developed a blinding headache, and the husband remembered that their ancient gas stove, which he had repaired for the occasion, had been causing similar problems of late from carbon monoxide leaking into the room. Looking about the healthiest of anyone, the baby responded almost instantaneously to a single dose of CARBO VEG. 30, while the rest of us took considerably longer to recover.

In chronic venous insufficiency and other forms of peripheral vascular disease, deoxygenation with coldness and bluish discoloration can analogously result from poor circulation and inadequate perfusion of the tissues.

In either case, despite feeling cold to the touch, CARBO VEG. patients generally want cold air to breathe, preferably blown on or near them for maximum exposure, and fan themselves vigorously if they are able.

With deoxygenation also a cardinal feature of the dying process, CARBO VEG. is known as "the corpse-reviver" because of its power to prolong life even in terminally ill patients to the point that wills, farewells, and other final arrangements can be made. For the newborn with respiratory distress and persistent cyanosis, CARBO VEG. can actually save life and prevent irreversible brain damage.

> Case 6.26. After a very fast labor, a woman of 36 gave birth to her fourth child with the cord wrapped tightly around the neck, thick meconium in the amniotic sac, and weak respiratory effort. One dose of CARBO VEG. 30 quickly revived this otherwise healthy newborn before we had a chance to suction her.

2. Indigestion, Gas, and Bacterial Action

Often associated with overgrowth of the gas-producing organisms of the intestinal flora, the deoxygenated CARBO VEG. state may also arise from overeating or indigestion from spoiled or excessively rich food. With activated charcoal still widely used in medicine for the symptomatic relief of belching or flatulence, the digestive symptoms of CARBO VEG. are almost always accompanied by gaseous distention and relieved by passing gas in either direction. CARBO VEG. patients are also given to overindulgence in the same rich sauces, gravies, and desserts that tend to make them ill.

> Case 6.27. Complaining primarily of water retention, a woman of 33 dated her problem to a big party the previous year, when overeating and subsequent food

poisoning resulted in an outbreak of hives that took
over a month to clear and had left her feeling below par
ever since. Although on a "starvation" diet when I saw
her, she was was also overly fond of rich foods and
sauces and would bloat up instantly after eating them.
Generally at her worst in hot, humid weather, she
wanted fresh, cold air blowing on her while she slept.
After CARBO VEG. 200, three doses in 24 hours, she
reported feeling better than she had in years, soon
becoming pregnant with her second child and having a
successful home birth without any difficulty.

3. Miscellaneous Symptoms

With undernourished blood and weakened blood vessels, patients
in need of CARBO VEG. are prone to nosebleeds or excessive
bleeding from wounds, with the menstrual period, or after birth or
miscarriage. Likewise, the gums may appear spongy or purple and
bleed easily; wounds are slow to heal and apt to become infected;
and the ankles are often bluish and swollen and subject to varicose
ulcers. On history and physical examination the overall impression
is one of sluggishness, stagnation, and failure to respond or heal in
a timely or vigorous fashion. Many conditions calling for CARBO
VEG. are aggravated in hot, humid weather.

4. Therapeutics

A leading remedy for rescue of the newborn, CARBO VEG. is
most helpful when the baby is deeply or persistently cyanotic but
making some efforts to breathe. In this situation, CARBO VEG. 30
may be given every few minutes if necessary.

When the symptoms agree, it is also a wonderful remedy for
miscellaneous complaints of pregnancy, such as overeating, indigestion, or venous stasis (varicose veins, hemorrhoids, etc.), with
the typical air hunger and desire to be fanned.

Case 6.28. Five months pregnant with her third child,
a woman of 28 became uncomfortably gassy after meals
and during sleep, when she felt as if she had eaten too

much and had to burp a lot and feel cold air blowing on her for relief. Previously fond of seconds even when feeling full, since becoming pregnant she had already disciplined herself against overindulgence with the prospect of even more dire consequences. CARBO VEG. 30 twice daily quickly relieved her distress, and she completed the pregnancy and gave birth successfully at home without further trouble.

With similar indications, CARBO VEG. may be useful after the birth for delayed recovery from Caesarean section or post-partum infection or indeed following any prolonged or debilitating illness.

CHAPTER 7

Seven Universal Remedies

The remedies in this chapter are used mostly in the treatment of chronic illness, and their symptom-pictures are much richer and fuller than can reasonably be compressed into a few paragraphs or easily mastered without considerable study and experience. Furthermore, their therapeutic range encompasses all organs and tissues and is by no means limited primarily to women's health. On the other hand, they are also useful in acute situations, and they raise issues so fundamental to health and so widely applicable to pregnancy and childbirth that it seemed imperative to attempt a brief introduction to them here.

SULPHUR

Trituration of elemental sulfur, brimstone, flowers of sulfur, S.

Often called the "king" of the *materia medica*, SULPHUR has produced and cured a greater diversity of symptoms than any other remedy, simulating virtually every known illness. It therefore became the keystone of Hahnemann's concept of the chronic diseases, and is still given as an intercurrent remedy when a more distinctive picture is lacking, often realigning the symptoms and pointing to the next remedy more clearly.

1. *Yin and Yang: Heat and Energy Phenomena*

The element sulfur is an essential component of all proteins and thus of all living matter. In the human body, high-energy sulfur bonds are the "business" end of insulin and Coenzyme A, which generate energy from the breakdown of carbohydrates and fats, respectively. Sulfur thus plays a pivotal role in the metabolic "furnace" wherein our body heat is produced and maintained. The great tradition of Chinese and Japanese medicine still identifies this energy with *ch'i*, the quintessential "stuff" of life itself.

Both the general style and particular symptoms of SULPHUR tend to revolve around excessive or unregulated heat production in some form. SULPHUR patients are generally overheated, tending to go about scantily clad in winter and cooling their feet down by putting them out of the blankets at night or walking around barefoot whenever possible. Nor do they tolerate heat well, especially hot rooms, hot baths, and warm blankets, although they may enjoy working or playing in the sun or sweating from a good workout. Despite often slovenly personal habits, they are sources of heat and vitality to everyone around them.

The same Yang quality is often noticeable in the temperament as well. SULPHUR children are natural leaders, aggressive and bossy yet popular with their followers. SULPHUR adults are apt to make excellent salesmen or eccentrics, ardently promoting their own opinions into causes of universal import and seldom taking "no" for an answer. Their bullying and insensitivity can sometimes be crudely destructive by igniting the ambitions or disregarding the frailties and sensibilities of others.

> *Case 7.1.* A two-year-old girl was brought in for "behavior problems." From the first she dominated the interview with sheer excess of vitality, which no matter how often restrained would quickly erupt again, without meanness or forethought, like some elemental force of nature. Ruddy-faced and overheated, she slept uncovered at night and ran around barefoot on the cold floor in the middle of winter. She was also in the midst of her "terrible twos," defiantly insisting on getting her

way and ever ready to throw a screaming fit on the floor if refused or contradicted. After SULPHUR 1M, three doses in 24 hours, she behaved as if her carburetor had been turned down a few notches, keeping shoes and blankets on, with fewer tantrums and a more agreeable disposition. Over the ensuing two years, she would come back for another dose of the remedy every six months or so, seldom needing any others.

2. Itching and Skin Eruptions

In accordance with Hering's Laws of Cure, SULPHUR ailments often originate in or discharge through the skin and the body surface. SULPHUR is an important remedy for skin eruptions of all kinds, particularly with itching and burning that are aggravated by heat, after a bath, or in bed at night.

> Case 7.2. Six weeks after an easy first birth, a 35-year-old woman complained of a patchy dryness and roughness of the skin, which after washing dishes, bathing, or getting warm in bed would blossom into an annoying, itchy rash that kept her awake most of the night. She felt quite well otherwise and was nursing her baby without any problems. SULPHUR 200, three doses in 24 hours, was all she needed to correct this typical complaint which she had had many times in the past.

SULPHUR is also used for internal complaints traceable to suppression of skin conditions in the past. Generally sensitive to soaps and often looking unclean even after a bath or shower, the skin tends to have a rough or uneven texture and may be subject to impetigo, boils, or pustules from time to time, as if needing to discharge impurities from within.

3. Miscellaneous Keynotes

Many SULPHUR complaints likewise have a certain "rough," crude, or uneven quality perhaps similarly related to irregularities in the heat mechanism. Thus the general overheating may bypass the relative coldness of certain parts or be punctuated by intervals of generalized chilliness. Depletion of ordinarily abundant energy reserves may lead to periods of exhaustion, typically around 11 A.M. Even the personality is uneven, tending to harp on the "big things" at the expense of details and nuances and alternating between ebullient and dispirited phases.

The appetite may be excessive, particularly for carbohydrates, sweets, and highly salted or hot, spicy foods, with a prodigious thirst for cold drinks, including beer and alcohol in all forms. The skin and mucous membranes of the nose, mouth, anus, vagina, and urethra are easily reddened and inflamed, while the pains of SULPHUR, which may occur anywhere in the body, are also typically burning in character and relieved by cold.

> *Case 7.3.* Seven months pregnant with her second child, a woman of 33 developed a clear vaginal discharge with severe itching and burning whenever she washed or urinated or made love. Otherwise her health was good, with no other complaints except a feeling of general malaise and discomfort in the heat, a tremendous thirst for ice-cold drinks, and a craving for hot, spicy foods that was equally unusual for her. After SULPHUR 200, the vaginitis and heat symptoms quickly receded, and the birth followed without difficulty two months later.

4. Therapeutics

SULPHUR is an important remedy in late pregnancy, when the dramatically increased blood volume tends to be associated with excessive heat production and other symptoms referable to it, notably edema, hypertension, insomnia, and the like.

> *Case 7.4.* In the final month of her third pregnancy a 31-year-old woman came in hugely swollen and uncomfortable. With a colorful history that included gonorrhea acquired on her wedding night and two episodes of hepatitis from intravenous drug use, she had had one successful home birth but still consumed 10–15 cigarettes and at least two glasses of wine daily without any pretense of concern. Her legs and feet were

markedly swollen and red, particularly in the heat, and she felt overheated and uncomfortable from heat in any form. Yet she seemed quite well otherwise and full of her usual insouciance and boisterous good humor.
SULPHUR 200 provoked a massive diuresis that lasted for several days and greatly relieved her swelling and discomfort. She gave birth easily three weeks later.

SULPHUR is also indispensable for minor complaints of pregnancy (hemorrhoids, vaginitis, eczema, etc.) associated with typical SULPHUR heat phenomena, and for babies and children after repeated acute illnesses or during convalescence.
ACONITE, ARNICA, PULSATILLA, and NUX VOMICA are complementary.

CALCAREA CARBONICA
Trituration of the middle layer of oyster shells, mostly calcium carbonate, $CaCO_3$.

1. *Infancy and Childhood: Delayed Growth and Development*
Hydroxides, phosphates, and carbonates of calcium are important components in the structural matrix of bones and teeth and thus play a pivotal role in the process by which infants and children acquire definite form and shape. As the basic constitutional remedy of early childhood, CALCAREA CARBONICA also addresses the "child" in older people, those features of physiognomy and aspects of character that, however fixed they may appear, are never complete and continue to develop throughout life.

In babies many CALCAREA CARBONICA characteristics reflect delay or deficiency in normal developmental processes (e.g., teething, walking, talking). Babies needing CALC. CARB. may be flabby and sometimes floppy, awkward, and poorly coordinated with undefined or blunted features or an overly cautious temperament.

Case 7.5. A 16-month-old girl was brought in because of developmental retardation. Born full-term by repeat Caesarean section, she had good Apgar scores but never learned to nurse vigorously and did not sit up or crawl until nine and thirteen months of age, respectively. When I saw her, she was still sleeping all night and most of the day and appeared to be slightly retarded mentally as well. Apart from a sweaty head and seemingly inexhaustible cravings for cheese, milk, and eggs, she showed few other symptoms, although the parents had noticed that her overall vitality and development suffered a clear setback after each DPT vaccination. One month after CALC. CARB. 10M, three doses in 24 hours, her mother reported accelerated progress in walking and talking. After four months she could walk by herself and talked quite well but still seemed a little slower and more immature than her contemporaries. At this point the remedy was repeated with even better effect, the mother reporting marked improvement in alertness, energy, and motor co-ordination to a level appropriate for her age.

On the other hand, CALC. CARB. children also tend to be cheerful and placid by nature, diligent and methodical in school and at play, and well able to retain what they learn. Indeed, they can easily become attached or fixated to a particular form once mastered and obstinately resistant to change not yet accepted or willed.

2. Chronicity: Protracted, Recurrent, and Relapsing Complaints

Illnesses calling for CALC. CARB. similarly tend to be protracted, slow to resolve, and subject to frequent recurrences and relapses. In adults, these background characteristics often go unnoticed until the failure of more obvious remedies forces a change of approach. CALC. CARB. thus addresses the underlying constitutional susceptibility to fall ill in certain ways and ultimately the problem of chronicity itself.

Case 7.6. An 11-month-old baby girl was brought in because of colds and URI's that had recurred all winter and never resolved, leaving a chronic residue of minor symptoms like thick, yellow nasal discharge, rattling in the chest, irregular bowels, and persistent diaper rash. Occasionally she would develop an acute illness with high fever that would respond to BELLADONNA, but something always remained. After a bout of premature labor arrested with alcohol, in the end the birth was three weeks late, the baby weighed nine pounds, and it took the mother over four hours to push her out. Slow to grasp the nipple or master the technique of nursing, she also seemed clumsy in crawling and walking and sweated profusely from her oversized head. Although a very "good" baby, she could not sleep without the breast in her mouth and often screamed when put down for a nap. Within a few days after a round of CALC. CARB. 200, her nose stopped running, the rattling disappeared, and her general health and development remained excellent for the rest of the winter.

3. Miscellaneous Keynotes

Often overweight and sweaty even after minimal effort, particularly on the head and face, children or adults needing CALC. CARB. also tend to be chilly and sensitive to sudden changes in the weather, especially to cold, wet weather, which makes them stiff, achy, or prone to colds or swollen glands. In many cases there are strong cravings for eggs, milk, and cheese, not infrequently with inability to tolerate them as well.

4. Therapeutics

The great constitutional remedy of babies and small children, CALC. CARB. can facilitate healthy development and nutrition even when no acute illness is present. It is often suggested by a number of chronic and seemingly unrelated or minor complaints such as thrush, cradle cap, or recurrent colds or ear infections, at which time the underlying nutritional and developmental themes are easily discerned. In such cases, CALC. CARB. 30 may be tried morning and night for three days at a time and repeated on a weekly basis as needed.

Case 7.7. A three-year-old girl had taken antibiotics several times each winter for recurrent ear infections. She had also had croup two weeks before her visit and often awoke in the night screaming from foot cramps. Weighing nine pounds at birth, she was still big and heavy for her age, but her muscles lacked definition and her speech and movements seemed awkward. Yet she was also intelligent, good-natured, and surprisingly dexterous with her hands. Her main problem was cold, wet weather, when she caught most of her colds and often ear infections as well. Apart from her DPT shots, she seldom ran a fever when ill, perspired mostly on her forehead, and had persistent cravings for milk, cheese, and eggs. After one round of CALC. CARB. 1M, her muscular development and co-ordination improved dramatically, and she got through the winter with no ear infections and one cold.

BELLADONNA and RHUS TOX. are complementary.

LYCOPODIUM

Tincture of spores or fresh plant, *Lycopodium clavatum*, N. O. Lycopodiaceae, club moss.

Used in the nineteenth century to make pills, LYCOPODIUM is another seemingly inert substance whose medicinal properties became apparent only after being prepared homeopathically. Like CALCAREA CARBONICA, its underlying themes are chronic and easily missed within the narrow perspective of a single illness. Its principal symptoms also seem unconnected in the sense that they have never been satisfactorily accounted for within a single explanatory framework.

1. Bilateral Asymmetry

Many LYCOPODIUM symptoms are one-sided, and most are predominantly right-sided or begin on the right side and proceed from right to left. When applicable to other seemingly unrelated symptoms as well, the same asymmetry may be used to describe the energy condition of the patient as a whole. Lateralizing symptoms often have special importance in homeopathy, precisely because they have nothing to do with the abstract pathological diagnosis, referring solely to the unique energy condition of the patient.

> *Case 7.8.* A 22-year-old college student consulted me for intermittent pain in the right ovary for the past seven months, especially around the time of ovulation and before her periods. She also had right-sided headaches and pain and tenderness under her right ribs that radiated into the groin and thigh. Described as "jabbing like sharp spikes," the groin pain kept her from sitting or bending over and was at its worst before and after exams, from the intense pressure she felt to excel academically; when her husband was away, which made her feel lonely and insecure; and from overeating or indigestion. No cyst was ever found. She often felt vaguely apprehensive at 4 P.M. but rarely at night unless she was home alone. A round of LYCOPODIUM 1M was given around midcycle, and a week later her pain was worse, involving the left ovary as well, and accompanied by facial neuralgia which also moved from right to left. LYCOPODIUM 10M was then given, and the pain gradually subsided, as did the whole obscure syndrome of right-sided symptoms and indigestion.

2. Circadian Variations

Another peculiar feature of many LYCOPODIUM illnesses is their tendency to worsen at certain hours of the day, chiefly in the late afternoon from 4 to 8 P.M. and in the morning on waking. When applicable to a group of otherwise unrelated symptoms, this pattern may also define the LYCOPODIUM symptom-picture as a whole. No less than its sidedness, the peculiar time aggravations of LYCOPODIUM tend to operate at a deeper level than can be attributed to any particular illness and thus hint at other important factors unseen or withheld.

3. Anxiety, Fear, and Hypochondriasis

The similarly asymmetrical and divisive mental and emotional picture is even more apt to confuse or mislead in this way. Often rather cerebral and unemotional and even cold and calculating about their own self-interest, chronic LYCOPODIUM patients also tend to be highly selective about what or how much to divulge about their inner lives. Indeed, their obsession to be in control may condemn them to an inner loneliness and isolation they cannot escape, their confident air and competent reputation concealing all too well the fear of inadequacy or failure that haunts them with every new challenge. One of the great remedies of ego-development, LYCOPODIUM corresponds to ailments trapped within the universal problems of cowardice and courage.

> *Case 7.9.* A 27-year-old attorney consulted me for palpitations. With a history of tachycardia and "fluttery" feelings in the chest since the age of 16, she had taken digitalis and other drugs for years until stopping all medications because of their side effects and her desire to get pregnant. Since then she had been even more nervous: her hands shook visibly, she could feel her heart pounding, and her resting pulse averaged 110 per minute. When she did become pregnant, her blood pressure shot up to the point that she decided to abort rather than risk it. Although inhibited and insecure around other lawyers in "high-pressure" situations and also generally more symptomatic at those times, she was then engaged in historic litigation on behalf of industrial workers seeking damages against the Federal Government. Typically at her worst after eating and in the late afternoon around 4 P.M., she liked to take walks in the fresh air for relief. After three doses of LYCOPODIUM 1M at midcycle, the trembling and palpitations rapidly subsided, followed by a series of right-sided symptoms which also passed, leaving her feeling more energetic, positive, and generally healthier than in a long time.

In acute illnesses, LYCOPODIUM patients may be overtly anxious, fearful, or hypochondriacal about their particular complaints, insisting that someone remain in the next room or nearby to be at their beck and call in case of trouble. Others may conceal the terror that motivates them by behaving tyrannically, or egotistically neglect to thank their helpers, tending to credit their own efforts first.

4. Miscellaneous Keynotes

Like the other constitutional remedies in this chapter, LYCOPODIUM can produce symptoms in every part of the body and helps to cure illnesses of every type. LYCOPODIUM patients are especially prone to abdominal discomfort from gaseous distention and may be relieved by burping or passing wind. With a tendency to crave sweets and an inordinately large appetite, they may also fill up quickly and are often extremely sensitive to overeating. When acutely ill, they usually prefer to avoid cold food and drinks in favor of hot or warm, which relieves their sore throats and many other symptoms. On the other hand, they are apt to feel "stuffy" in overheated rooms and to want cool, fresh air.

5. Therapeutics

LYCOPODIUM is an important remedy in women's health. It has an affinity for the ovaries, particularly the right, and many symptoms are aggravated before the menstrual period. With the usual indications (right-sided, late afternoon aggravations, bloating, anxiety, etc.), it has also been useful in the treatment of premenstrual syndrome (PMS).

> Case 7.10. A woman of 25 consulted me for ovarian pain. Since her appendectomy two years ago, she had suffered from a sharp, burning pain in her right ovary, typically from ovulation until the period. Often worse from movement or exercise, it could sometimes be relieved by making love or doing something enjoyable to distract herself. In spite of being supported comfortably by her father, her literary ambitions continued to be overshadowed by fear and insecurity

about not having a career or job or money of her own. Passionately in love with the classics, she lived with the man who had been her favorite professor in college. Usually tired and cranky by 4 P.M., she would often perk up again in the evening, avoiding large meals and cold drinks and coveting the time she spent by herself. After LYCOPODIUM 1M at midcycle and a brief right-to-left headache, her ovarian pain was greatly relieved and slowly receded into the background. Repeat doses were given at rare intervals, and she remained well.

LYCOPODIUM is also useful in headaches, indigestion, sore throats, and other acute complaints of pregnant and nursing women, particularly when right-sided and aggravated by overeating or cold food or relieved by warm drinks. In such cases, LYCOPODIUM 30 may be tried four times daily as needed. It is a wonderful remedy for children as well. But mainly it is used for chronic complaints.

> *Case 7.11.* Seven months pregnant with her second child, a woman of 30 consulted me for varicose veins which were swollen and painful late every afternoon and only on the right side. Although she had had no problems with her first birth and as a nurse felt more secure in the hospital environment, she was determined to try a home birth. Still terrified of heights, she had recurrent "stress" dreams of watching someone falling from a cliff. One dose of LYCOPODIUM 200 gave her profound relief, and a second one month later helped her to finish the pregnancy with only minor discomfort, although she needed an emergency C-section for a ten-pound baby with a face presentation.

LACHESIS is complementary.

LACHESIS

Trituration of the venom, *Lachesis muta muta*, N. O. Ophidia, bushmaster or Surukuku.

LACHESIS is made from the venom of the deadly bushmaster snake, which lives in the Amazon jungle and often attains a length of ten feet or more. The name comes from the three Greek goddesses of Fate, who fix the span of life: Clotho, who spins the thread; Lachesis, who draws it out to its appointed length; and Atropos, who cuts it. History records that the great Constantine Hering, who contributed the first proving of LACHESIS venom, died on the anniversary of the event fifty-two years later, almost to the day.[1]

LACHESIS belongs to the rattlesnake family (Crotalidae), the poisons of which coagulate and hemolyze the blood and may compromise its circulation to the heart, brain, and vital organs. A superb remedy with important applications to gynecology and every other branch of medicine, LACHESIS is famous for its vivid and often unmistakable keynote symptoms, although no unifying interpretation of them has ever been wholly satisfactory.

1. Bilateral Asymmetry

Many Crotalid venoms produce asymmetric or one-sided disturbances of the bioenergetic field, but none more so than LACHESIS, whose symptoms are markedly skewed to the left or at least tend to start on the left and proceed from left to right. In this respect it is the mirror-image of LYCOPODIUM, which is also complementary to it.

> Case 7.12. A 39-year-old woman consulted me for bursting premenstrual headaches radiating back from the left eyebrow and relieved by cold washcloths. During the week before her period she was also notably tense and irritable and subject to frequent lower back pain and sciatica, likewise on the left side. All of her symptoms typically vanished at the start of her menstrual flow, which tended to be heavy and clotted. In the habit of stretching out her turtlenecks until they hung loosely, she could not bear tight clothing of any kind around her waist or throat. After a round of LACHESIS 1M at midcycle and LACHESIS 12 as needed

for headache, she needed the remedy only twice more, once during her typical autumn sinusitis and again a year after our first meeting, practically to the day.

2. Sleep Disturbances

LACHESIS often interferes with the sleep process in a most profound and remarkable way. Unlike people with insomnia who simply cannot fall asleep, LACHESIS patients instinctively resist sleep because it seems to do them harm. In many cases, their symptoms are intensified during or after sleep, such that they are likely to feel progressively worse the longer they remain unconscious. Others may resist even getting ready for sleep or wake up with a start when they begin to drift off, as though intolerant of the sleep process itself.

> *Case 7.13.* A woman of 33 consulted me for vertigo, which two years ago had roused her from sleep with the sensation that she was falling out of bed as she tried to turn over. Since then it often recurred on looking up or turning her head but most intensely as she opened her eyes after sleep, when she also felt "fuzzy" in the head and her eyeballs seemed to oscillate back and forth involuntarily. After normal hearing tests an ear specialist detected cochlear otosclerosis in her left ear. Otherwise she was in good health, although curiously intolerant of tight clothing and hot, humid weather. After a round of LACHESIS 1M at midcycle, her dizziness subsided and did not reappear, and she felt more energetic and positive, sleeping normally and requiring no further treatment.

3. Choking and Constriction from Touch, Pressure, and Tight Clothing

With a particular affinity for the throat, LACHESIS often benefits patients with choking sensations that are aggravated during sleep, on waking, or from the pressure of something worn snugly around the neck, such as a tie or scarf. Similar constricting sensations are common in the head, extremities, chest, heart, lungs, and abdominal and pelvic organs, which are analogously sensitive to pressure from tight clothing, such as a hat or waistband. In sinus headaches or earaches, the overlying skin may be abnormally sensitive to touch as well, and even a soft caress can be most unwelcome. LACHESIS patients are also subject to headaches or earaches from exposure to cold wind or from swimming or diving and the pressure of water inside the ear. In general, sensations of constriction internally tend to be matched by sensitivity to touch and pressure on the outside.

4. *Internal Tension Relieved by an External Discharge*

Underlying much of the symptom-picture of LACHESIS is the analogous pattern of internal tension and external release. Not only muscular or nervous tension, which may occur anywhere in the body, and the peculiar constrictive sensations already described, but many other symptoms of LACHESIS as well are likely to be relieved by some external secretion, elimination, or discharge and brought on or aggravated when the corresponding outlet is blocked.

In adult women, such a mechanism is regularly provided by the menstrual cycle, at the end of which accumulated energy blocks are released and hormonal batteries recharged. LACHESIS is a leading remedy for premenstrual syndrome, in which symptoms build and peak before the flow and release abruptly once it is established, and also for menopause or amenorrhea, when further health problems may develop from closure of or interference with this important escape-valve.

> *Case 7.14.* A woman of 49 consulted me for a recurrence of systemic lupus erythematosus (SLE), which had blossomed four years earlier, following a total hysterectomy for fibroid tumors and subsequent estrogen replacement. Her chief symptoms were marked fatigue, sore throat and burning in the stomach and intestines, mouth ulcers, throbbing pains in the left arm, shoulder, and knee, and persistent earache, also left-sided. Although her pains were generally worse during sleep, she slept badly even without them and would sometimes

awaken bolt upright in the process of losing consciousness. Other symptoms included swelling of the eyes in the sun and faulty concentration, which greatly hindered her career as a professional writer. Much preferring the cold, she could not tolerate hot, humid weather, and reacted violently to alcohol and conventional drugs. LACHESIS 1M and 10M in very infrequent doses has helped keep this woman in splendid health for over five years.

LACHESIS patients also tend to talk a lot to express or relieve tension more than to converse or communicate and can spit out monologue in a rapid-fire chatter that almost trips over syllables in its haste to expel them. If LACHESIS has one central theme, it is this powerful drive to release internal tension through some sort of expressive discharge.

5. Tissue Affinities

Like all the Crotalid venoms, LACHESIS has a special affinity for the blood and circulation and tends to be useful for both hemor-rhagic and thrombotic phenomena, including heart attack, stroke, purpura, hemolytic anemia, functional uterine bleeding, and the like. There may be purplish or ecchymotic discoloration of the skin or signs of venous congestion like hemorrhoids or varices, e.g., in alcoholism, for which the remedy is particularly useful.

Another major target area is the crowded region of the head and face that includes the throat, ears, and sinuses, all highly sen-sitive to touch and pressure, including wind, storms, and abrupt changes in barometric pressure as indicated above. LACHESIS patients are exceedingly vulnerable to sinus headaches, earaches, sore throats, and nosebleeds, all of which are aggravated in hot, humid weather and of course relieved by discharging whatever secretions may be present.

6. Miscellaneous Symptoms

Warm or chilly, LACHESIS patients usually prefer fresh air and are intolerant of hot, humid weather. Particularly before or during the period, their sexual energy is often very strong and the genitals themselves may be extremely sensitive to a snug-fitting tampon or speculum. Emotionally they can be haughty, irritable, and possessive, especially before the period, and given to passionate outbursts of anger, jealousy, or sadness.

7. *Therapeutics*

LACHESIS is indispensable in gynecology. Widely useful in the treatment of PMS, amenorrhea, and menstrual disorders of all kinds, it is also a leading remedy for complaints of the menopause. With a decided affinity for the ovaries, particularly the left, it has helped many patients afflicted with endometriosis when the typical elements are present. In pregnancy, it is useful for such common congestive problems as hypertension, hemorrhoids, varicose veins, ovarian pain, sore throats, sinus headaches, and earaches. When indicated in such cases, LACHESIS 30 may be tried up to every few hours as needed. It should also be considered for rescue of the newborn and for vaccine-related illnesses in babies and small children.

> *Case 7.15.* Seven months pregnant with her first child, a 31-year-old woman had had a severe cough for three weeks and still produced quantities of blood-streaked sputum along with considerable fatigue and exhaustion. The cough was especially severe during the night, waking her up frequently and getting worse the more she slept. Her other complaints were heartburn after sweets or alcohol and a stitching pain under the left ribs when she sat up. After three doses of LACHESIS 200 the cough cleared up within 24 hours, and she kept fit and healthy for the rest of the pregnancy, giving birth at home without any complications.

LYCOPODIUM is complementary.

ARSENICUM ALBUM

Trituration of arsenious trioxide, $As_2 O_3$.

1. *Fatigue, Exhaustion, and Restlessness*

Arsenic is poisonous to all living cells, and the most important symptoms of ARSENICUM are much as would be expected in an organism sapped and devitalized by some noxious substance or from the toxic wastes of its own internal decomposition. Thus ARSENICUM patients typically suffer from profound fatigue and prostration disproportionate to any effort, often needing to rest after walking downstairs or feeling faint or dizzy after a minor exertion such as a bowel movement. Yet they cannot sit still or find any relief from movement, as if condemned to a futile quest for the inner peace that alone could quiet them.

2. *Coldness and Lack of Vital Heat; Burning Pains Relieved by Heat*

Another hallmark of the debilitated ARSENICUM state is a profound coldness that seems to permeate every cell. Almost invariably chilly and aggravated by the cold, ARSENICUM patients appreciate fur coats and overheated rooms, and most of their symptoms are benefited by hot drinks or heat in any form. Even the ubiquitous burning pains are paradoxically relieved by heat, again suggestive of poisoning or auto-intoxication at the cellular level.

3. *Insecurity: Fear, Anxiety, Obsessive-Compulsive Behavior*

In much the same way, the mental and emotional symptoms of patients needing ARSENICUM ALBUM are often colored by an unnaturally heightened awareness of having been poisoned by something at the cellular level that cannot be healed. The overt symptoms that they complain of may thus be overshadowed, intensified, or even heralded by a deep existential anguish or a conscious fear of death and decay that can be temporarily assuaged but never entirely overcome.

Indeed, many ARSENICUM ailments originate on the psychic level with a fear of being alone or an obsessive elaboration of purely subjective symptoms that demands continual reassurance and can monopolize the time and energy of anyone willing to help. In more advanced or chronic cases, ARSENICUM patients may become compulsively orderly about details of dress, decor, or outward form, as if trying to contain the process of disintegration within.

> *Case 7.16.* A 43-year-old graduate student with allergic asthma was using inhalers and bronchodilators regularly, often for weeks at a time. Around cats, dust, mold, and in cold, damp weather, her post-nasal drip would turn into wheezing and a tight, productive cough that tended to wake her in the wee hours of the morning. Afraid to be alone at such times, she prayed for someone to hold her and keep her warm with hot drinks and tender solicitude. With furrowed brow and groping fingers, she qualified each detail with the utmost precision and delicacy, as if to strike a balance between the urgency of her need and the etiquette of polite conversation. ARSENICUM ALBUM 1M was given at midcycle, along with ARSENICUM ALBUM 30 as needed. In the three years since then, apart from occasional refills and one bad attack on the eve of her doctoral exams, she has needed little else.

4. Miscellaneous Keynotes

One of the great periodic remedies, ARSENICUM can be helpful for symptoms that recur weekly, fortnightly, annually on the same date, or at regular intervals, when the characteristic indications are present. Many patients report special times of aggravation around twilight, just after midnight, or in the wee hours of the morning. Also splendid for colds, hay fever, allergies, and catarrhal inflammation of the mucous membranes generally, ARSENICUM is especially indicated for acrid, sour, corrosive, offensive, or bloody discharges from the nose, throat, rectum, or vagina.

> *Case 7.17.* Thirty-five weeks pregnant with her second child, a woman of 30 developed severe hay fever with sore, "vulnerable" sensations in her ribs, paralyzing

fatigue, and a hoarse cough provoked by the least exposure to cold air or wind. Tormented most of all by a dry
throat and itchy palate, she was reduced to sipping a ther-
mos of hot lemonade which she never let out of her sight.
With the help of ARSENICUM ALBUM 30 four times
daily, her hay fever cleared in a few days and never came
back. She had a successful home birth six weeks later.

ARSENICUM is also important for the treatment of gastroenteritis, food poisoning, colitis, and other illnesses with nausea,
vomiting, and diarrhea. Many different ailments calling for it are
accompanied by a burning thirst, especially for warm drinks and
small sips at a time.

Case 7.18. Previously in good health, a 26-year-old
woman developed abdominal cramps and watery
diarrhea. For three days her movements were small and
very frequent, streaked with mucus or blood, and
followed by feelings of urging, straining, and never being
finished. Too exhausted to report for work, where several
colleagues had recently taken ill in similar fashion, she
was too nauseated to eat, and only sips of peppermint tea
gave her temporary relief. Although shivering with cold
and wrapped in heavy blankets, she had no fever, and
her stool exam and culture were negative. On
ARSENICUM ALBUM 200 four times daily, she made a
speedy recovery and was back at work in a few days.

5. *Therapeutics*

Invaluable for acute and chronic illnesses of every type,
ARSENICUM has power over every organ and tissue in the body.
A superb remedy for food poisoning, gastroenteritis, and dysentery,
it is equally applicable in bronchial asthma, hay fever, colds, and
allergies of the respiratory tract when the characteristic symptom-picture is present.

It is a leading remedy for chronic, debilitating illnesses like
metastatic cancer and for the final stages of the dying process
with auto-intoxication and typical ARSENICUM features. It can

be lifesaving for severely depressed newborn infants with or without meconium aspiration. In such cases, ARSENICUM 30 may have to be given as often as every 30 seconds together with conventional methods of resuscitation.

> *Case 7.19.* At her home in the country, a 20-year-old woman gave birth to her first child, a girl of eight pounds, after a prolonged second stage. Her body covered with green meconium, the baby took one gasp and then breathed no more. Brisk suctioning produced more thick meconium, and I was unable to intubate or even visualize the trachea. By now the child was limp, white, and motionless with a heartbeat of 60 per minute, responding feebly to mouth-to-mouth resuscitation but unable to breathe on her own. I put a tiny bit of ARSENICUM ALBUM 200 on her tongue, and she awoke with a jolt, crying and flailing, her heartbeat vigorous at 140 per minute and her skin glowing pink with the flame of existence. The whole evolution took no more than a few seconds. After a night in the hospital to be on the safe side, she went home in the morning with no outward sign that anything unusual had happened. Experiences like these are inscribed for life in every practitioner's mind.

In pregnancy ARSENICUM is used mostly for nausea and vomiting, gastroenteritis, allergies, asthma, and other incidental complaints.

PHOSPHORUS

Saturated solution of elemental phosphorus in absolute alcohol or triturate of red amorphous phosphorus, P.

Phosphorus is indispensable to all life. Calcium phosphates form the chemical matrix of bones and teeth; high-energy phosphate bonds carry the energy allotments to the tissues; phospholipids form the myelin sheath and other substances required for nerve transmission; nucleic acid phosphates store genetic information inside cells and relay it to their offspring.

Elemental phosphorus, on the other hand, is highly toxic, producing cellular necrosis of the liver and hemorrhagic disorders of the blood and clotting mechanism. Patients needing PHOS-PHORUS tend to show signs and symptoms analogous to those of phosphorus poisoning and unnaturally heightened or exaggerated functioning in certain areas.

1. *Tissue Affinities*

As might be expected, PHOSPHORUS has proved useful in acute and chronic hepatitis, cirrhosis, and other liver diseases with deficiencies in prothrombin and other clotting factors, as well as in purpura and bleeding tendencies of all types. It is also an important remedy for chronic diseases with necrosis or destruction of bone, particularly the lower jaw, and for metastatic cancer generally. An equally important predisposition for the lower respiratory tract (lungs, bronchi, trachea, larynx) makes PHOSPHORUS a leading remedy in the treatment of lobar and bronchial pneumonia, bacterial or viral, and of acute and chronic tracheobronchitis, bronchitis, and laryngitis as well.

Especially well suited to tall, thin, frail, narrow-chested individuals with weak lungs and a history of bronchitis or pneumonia, PHOSPHORUS when indicated has helped both dry and productive coughs, typically worse around midnight, from talking or deep breathing, and often accompanied by laryngitis with hoarseness and bloody or rusty sputum.

> *Case 7.20.* Thirty-two weeks pregnant with her second child, a woman of 34 complained of a nasty cough and laryngitis that had lasted for over a week. Mostly dry and brassy, the cough tended to wake her in the night, when her right lower ribs hurt during the paroxysms and she would sometimes leak urine. In a voice barely more than a whisper she recounted the tale of her thirst, which impelled her to drink large volumes of ice water and to chew on cracked ice whenever possible. PHOSPHORUS 30 morning and night and as needed in between helped her to finish off this stubborn cough

126

within a few days, and she went on to have her baby at home without further difficulty and right on time.

2. Fear, Empathy, and Imagination

With its strong affinity for the brain and nervous system, PHOS-PHORUS tends to be very helpful for patients who suffer from excessively facile or uncontrolled flights of imagination or from mental or emotional excitement of any kind. As if their nerves were poorly insulated and unable to transmit impulses selectively, many PHOSPHORUS patients are capable of empathic or even telepathic overidentification with the feelings and sufferings of others and a corresponding inability to differentiate them from their own.

Often of artistic temperament and motivated to communicate with other people, patients needing this remedy tend to be easily frightened when left alone and prone to wild fears and fantasies such as spirits in the night, monsters under the water, or incurable diseases in their own bodies. Although easily comforted by a reassuring word or embrace, their fears may return in full force by night or as soon as the company has gone home.

Case 7.21. A 28-year-old woman was 26 weeks pregnant with her second child when she consulted me for fatigue and indigestion. As a child she had been hospitalized several times for pneumonia and pleurisy and at 25 had bled heavily for three months while on oral contraceptives. When I saw her, she complained mostly of palpitations that would force her to stop whatever she was doing and of feeling bloated and gassy at times, with heartburn from tomatoes and green peppers. Her hematocrit was 33.6 per cent. Soft-spoken and timid, she often looked to her husband to answer for her, and her eyes opened wide and filled with tears as she remembered a dream in which she had had to take her baby to the hospital "for inspection" and the doctors had criticized her and wanted to take the baby away. Always reassured by the affection and companionship of her husband, she could not seem to calm her fears when he was away. With the help of PHOSPHORUS 200 her anemia and palpitations quickly subsided, she felt stronger and more confident, and when her time came she had a beautiful home birth with no problems or complications.

3. Miscellaneous Keynotes

With or without the fear of thunder and lightning often reported by PHOSPHORUS patients, many particular symptoms of the remedy are likely to be aggravated before or during an electrical storm. Although hypersensitive to the slightest imaginative or emotional stimulation, these patients tend to appreciate companionship and physical affection and often improve from being rubbed or massaged. Ordinarily on the chilly side and rather sensitive to the cold, they may also be extremely thirsty for ice-cold drinks, intolerant of warm drinks, and subject to headaches and burning pains throughout the body that are relieved by cold.

4. Therapeutics

PHOSPHORUS can be useful for nausea and vomiting of pregnancy and for miscellaneous acute complaints of pregnant women like bronchitis, laryngitis, and herpes. When the typical indications are present, it should also be considered for acute hepatitis, bleeding gums, purpura, and other hemorrhagic disorders, including a history of repeated miscarriage or bleeding later in pregnancy or afterwards.

> *Case 7.22.* Eight weeks into her first pregnancy a 29-year-old woman was incapacitated by constant nausea and dry heaves, particularly on getting up in the morning. Sensitive to the smell and sight of food, she was relieved for a time by vomiting but could eat solid food only by washing it down with cold milk or ice-cold drinks, for which she was insatiably thirsty. In a loud, raucous banter, she effectively communicated her own fears and need for reassurance by her hilarious spoofing and poking fun at them. A history of gonorrhea, genital herpes, PID, and repeated vaginal infections also

inspired a number of bawdy tales. PHOSPHORUS 30 was given four times daily, and in less than two weeks her nausea was essentially gone. She remained healthy for the rest of the pregnancy, notwithstanding a recurrent herpes outbreak in the fourth month and a procession of classic pregnancy fears that often seemed exaggerated but always responded to patient listening and simple explanation. No other remedies were given, and she gave birth normally after a strong, spirited, and beautiful labor that did us all proud.

PHOSPHORUS is also a superb remedy for fears, coughs, "growing pains," and other miscellaneous complaints of children, usually with a prominent imaginative or empathetic component.

Case 7.23. A lovely, wide-eyed girl of five was disturbed by a persistent fear of the dark and obsessive thoughts or fantasies such as hearing noises in the closet and imagining that someone was lurking there. Apart from the usual quota of colds and fevers, she seemed healthy enough and generally slept well, but scary movies were apt to result in nightmares, and nonsensical images like E.T. sporting a moustache regularly crowded into her mind and could not be erased. With a fear of thunder and a tendency to come down with high fevers at the approach of a storm, she was also intelligent, artistic, and almost telepathically sensitive to what others were feeling, often developing stomach aches as a result. Over the past two years, infrequent doses of PHOSPHORUS 1M and 10M have done wonders to help calm her fears and find creative paths for her gifted imagination.

NATRUM MURIATICUM
Trituration of sea salt, NaCl.

Salt or sodium chloride is essential for life, and a precise degree of salinity is indispensable for maintaining the osmotic pressure of the blood and body fluids and the integrity of the cells that live in them. Salt has been known since antiquity to preserve food from spoiling, and to flavor the tears of grief.

1. Ailments from Grief

NATRUM MUR. is even more difficult to describe concisely and to recognize in acute situations than the other remedies discussed in this chapter. Its underlying issues are so universal and its particular symptoms so vague or generic by comparison that even veteran homeopaths easily miss the forest for the trees or overprescribe the remedy on ideology alone.

Like IGNATIA, to which it is often complementary, NATRUM MURIATICUM is suitable for patients who are grieving or have suffered grievously in the past. But while IGNATIA expresses the nervous and emotional instability of acute grief, the pattern of NATRUM MUR. is one of chronic emotional and physiological rigidity established after repeated or habitual disappointment.

These themes are well summarized in the Biblical tale of Lot's wife, uprooted from her home and kindred, who cannot resist looking back as her homeland is destroyed by fire and her past reduced to ashes. For her human frailty the punishment seems excessively cruel: to survive as a pillar of salt, as if embalmed forever in mourning and remembrance.

Clinically, NATRUM MUR. patients need not be acutely depressed or even able to identify particular reasons for their unhappiness. Sometimes the only clue is a grim or joyless expression, a humorless attitude, or a rationale of futility and resignation that obviously goes back a very long time. At the same time, their admirable commitments to honesty, fairness, punctuality, and the fulfillment of interpersonal obligations can be too exacting or literal for anyone including themselves to accommodate or satisfy. Seldom allowing themselves to weep at all or at most only privately, NATRUM MUR. patients seem to have programmed themselves to resist the comfort and affection that they long for and to feel guilty or ashamed afterward for any relief obtained.

> Case 7.24. Suffering unremittingly from rheumatoid arthritis for 17 years, a woman of 52 had been maintained successfully on gold salts for most of that

time, although her joints continued to deteriorate and had required four arthroscopic surgeries. A course of bee venom injections had provoked a generalized aggravation of her condition that lasted for months and finally subsided only when further treatment with antimetabolites was recommended as the only alternative. Yet she had managed to complete her professional training, recovered well after each surgery, and was still working full-time despite severe pain and obvious disability. When I saw her, most of her limbs were affected, and her pains were mostly viselike and penetrating, typically aggravated by fatigue and relieved by warmth and rest, but not much affected by changes in weather or climate. The remainder of her history was dominated by grief, fear, and the quiet heroism of everyday life lived in the face of constant suffering. Abused by her father, molested by her aunt, and unheard by her mother, she found affection and safety only with her grandmother and had to put herself though college and graduate school, only to be stricken with a crippling disease. No longer able to practice her profession, she carried on as an administrator. Outcast as a lesbian by her family, she remained a true friend to many and had never been promiscuous in love. Slowly but surely over a period of many months with the help of two doses of NATRUM MUR. 1M, her pain and stiffness subsided, she regained strength in her hands and fingers, and her general energy and outlook improved to an extent that neither of us had realistically thought possible.

2. Miscellaneous Symptoms

NATRUM MUR. may be indicated for almost any ailment, and affect virtually any tissue or organ, in a context of unremitting or prolonged grief, sorrow, or disappointment and a clinical picture of rigidity or "stuckness" evocative of them. Thus, in addition to the typical discharge and irritation, the NATRUM MUR. hay fever might have an element of blockage or obstruction, or perhaps a sinus headache. Like most of its symptoms, these would tend to be intensified by direct sunlight and relieved by a cool washcloth. Although preferring in most cases to keep their rooms cool with access to fresh air, NATRUM MUR. patients are not necessarily warm-blooded and may be quite the opposite.

As might be expected, individuals needing this remedy are often strongly attracted to or intolerant of salt and salty foods, as well as the seashore, the salt air, the ocean, and the fish that live in it. As with IGNATIA and SEPIA, the symptoms of NATRUM MUR. are likely to be relieved by exercise if the patient is still capable of it.

> *Case 7.25.* Eight months pregnant with her third child, a 35-year-old woman came in complaining of nasal congestion and headache that made it difficult for her to sleep. As if I were somehow responsible for them, she threw her symptoms at me like an accusation, feeling very much alone and sorry for herself. Since their relocation from Florida a short time ago, her husband had not yet found work, which made her feel insecure and harshly critical of him. Yet she also insisted that they were getting along fine and that in any case their relationship was none of my business. Her particular symptoms were nondescript except for a marked craving for salt and a general improvement from exercise and being near the sea. After a round of NATRUM MUR. 1M was given without any obvious effect, I suggested NATRUM MUR. 30 three times daily for a while, and her headaches promptly subsided, her sleep improved, and she gave birth normally about a month later.

3. Therapeutics

NATRUM MUR. is indispensable in homeopathy and may be indicated under the most diverse circumstances and for ailments of every type. In pregnancy, it is useful for nausea and vomiting as well as headaches, colds, allergies, and gastrointestinal or other incidental complaints against a background of sorrow or disappointment with physical symptoms that seem to call attention to it. After labor, the remedy is equally valuable in the treatment of depression, fatigue, and other common postpartum complaints.

> *Case 7.26.* Eight weeks pregnant with her first child, a woman of 25 had been severely nauseated since the first week of conception. Much worse with her stomach empty, she ate larger meals and more often than ever before yet without interest in food except as a means of relief and nourishment. Only salty food consistently interested her. Her other complaints were increased nasal congestion and uterine pain at the time of intercourse. Actually she had not reached orgasm with her husband after the first six months of their relationship, when she had told him about her previous sexual experiences and the depth and coldness of his anger had frightened and shocked her. An only child, she had also been especially close and devoted to her father, who had died suddenly of a cerebral hemorrhage when she was thirteen. Except for a blood pressure of 135/95, she was otherwise in good health. NATRUM MUR. 200 twice daily gave her prompt and effective relief in a few days and did not have to be repeated. She completed the pregnancy and had a daughter at home without any further difficulty.

Seldom required for acute complaints and situations, NATRUM MUR. is usually given for more inveterate or chronic complaints that are apt to require experienced professional help. The public is nevertheless well advised to be familiar with it, since it may be indicated to remove obstacles to recovery and helps to demonstrate how illness both arises from the life energy and plays out into it as well.

> *Case 7.27.* A woman of 27 reported that her hay fever had become much more severe over the past three years since moving to the area at her husband's insistence and leaving behind her home, job, and friends. Her violent

and spiteful rages at that time brought back memories of her childhood, when her father had threatened her with a gun and she came down with colitis in the fourth grade from being repeatedly humiliated by her teacher in front of the class. By the time I saw her, she was divorced and had fallen in love with a married man. Her allergic symptoms included a stuffed nose, "blocked" sinuses, and gluey postnasal drip with some itching, all somewhat worse before a storm. A heavy smoker, she also suffered from menstrual cramps and depression and rejected all attempts to console her, since they made her feel weak, foolish, or inadequate. After a dose of NATRUM MUR. 200, she experienced a sense of well-being that she had not known for years, and after a brief aggravation her nose and sinuses cleared as well. When her symptoms returned in force some weeks later, she stormed out of my office rather than wait ten minutes past the time of her appointment. Soon after repeating the remedy, she telephoned to report that she felt much improved and very grateful.

IGNATIA and SEPIA are complementary.

PART III

Therapeutics

This final section is devoted to common problems of pregnancy, childbirth, and the newborn period, and to remedies particularly helpful for each, with illustrative cases wherever possible. In addition to those remedies previously discussed, others of more specialized interest will be introduced.

Because remedies should always be selected on the basis of the totality of symptoms, the list of possibilities for any given condition can never be complete, and others will certainly be needed. I have included only the remedies that I myself have used the most, in order to develop a basic methodology for finding the best one at the time. In many cases, further study will be required (see bibliography). Many complaints have been assigned to "early" and "late" pregnancy somewhat arbitrarily, since they may also occur at other times.

When considering remedies for a particular condition, students should first try to grasp the picture of the remedy as a whole, and not rely solely on the brief summaries provided in this section for remedies discussed more fully elsewhere.

CHAPTER 8

Early Pregnancy: First Trimester

Miscarriage and Infertility

Although often amenable to homeopathic care, established infertility, including inability to conceive and repeated miscarriage, lies beyond the scope of this book and calls for the help of a trained professional. Simple miscarriage, on the other hand, is a normal physiological process often requiring no treatment and carrying no prognostic implications for the future.

Contemporary research indicates that at least 10% of all pregnancies end in miscarriage,[1] quite often undiagnosed or at most suspected because of a slightly heavier period than usual. Such minor disturbances are particularly likely if the embryo dies in the first month, before obvious symptoms of pregnancy develop, and even more so in the first week, when it has not yet implanted and is still free-swimming. Since a suspected or feared pregnancy is also most easily prevented at this time, women have always used herbs like tansy or pennyroyal to keep the period on time.[2]

As the spontaneous termination of an unviable pregnancy with or without discernible labor, miscarriage is effectively complete once the embryo and other products of conception are expelled. After six weeks these can usually be seen as a small globular or gelatinous mass, quite distinct from the surrounding

blood, and often preceded or followed by membranes or fila-
mentous strands of placental tissue.

Today performed almost routinely, surgical dilatation and curet-
tage (D&C) is essentially a precaution to minimize the risk of
further bleeding and infection by removing all retained tissue
fragments. Once the embryo is passed and contractions and bleeding subside, the surgery may safely be omitted if the woman is
otherwise in good health and willing to be monitored carefully
for the next 48 hours or so.

Much as with labor, homeopathic care is indicated if the contractions are unduly prolonged or painful, the bleeding excessive
or unremitting, or the process is otherwise delayed or "stuck" at any
point. Remedies are especially useful in cases of threatened miscarriage, where the natural evolution is arrested in the earlier
stages before any tissue is passed, or after the fact, if painful contractions or bleeding persist. At such times, bleeding can be just as
insidious as after labor and may not be apparent clinically until
dangerous amounts of blood have been lost, so that close supervision is mandatory. Moreover, the remedies to be considered are
much the same as for abnormal or dysfunctional labor and postpartum bleeding. (See Chapters 10 and 11.)

1. CAULOPHYLLUM

This remedy should be considered when the contractions are
sharp and spasmodic, centered very low in the pelvis, and associated with excessive weakness, fatigue, and shaking, trembling, or
nervous excitement. In more advanced cases when miscarriage
fails to complete itself, products of conception may be retained,
often with cramping and bleeding as a result of uterine hypotonicity. CAULOPHYLLUM may also be tried preventively if the
woman has miscarried similarly in the past or if such a picture
seems imminent or threatening. (See Chapter 3.)

2. CIMICIFUGA

The symptoms indicating CIMICIFUGA are uterine dysfunction
accompanied by negativity, morbid fears, or evidence of fragmenting such as choreiform movements, alternating symptoms, and the

like. The remedy may also be given to prevent miscarriage with a history of this type in the past. It is equally useful for prevention and treatment of premature labor and other late-pregnancy complications associated with serious congenital defects. (See Chapter 3.)

> *Case 8.1.* A 24-year-old woman had been in good health until ten weeks into her second pregnancy, when the death of her father left her in control of the family home and business and aroused the resentment of her sister, who had not spoken to her since. At this point she began complaining of severe headaches that felt like a band around her head or "as if the top would come off" and usually made her dizzy and weak and disinclined to do anything but lie down and rest. Never prone to headaches in the past, she began to suspect that there was something wrong with the baby, noticing "weird" cramps low in the pelvis that would come and go quickly or alternate from side to side. With the aid of CIMICIFUGA 200, three doses in 24 hours, and CIMICIFUGA 12 every two hours as needed, she did indeed miscarry a week later, as she had foreseen, but with no problems or complications. Within four months she was pregnant again, this time carrying it through easily and giving birth at home without difficulty.

3. PULSATILLA

A leading remedy for miscarriage, PULSATILLA will usually be suggested by its general style (emotions too freely adaptable, physical symptoms ever-changing), together with typical keynotes — craving for fresh air, intolerance of warm rooms, overeating, rich foods, and the rest. (See Chapter 4.)

4. SEPIA

In threatened or incomplete miscarriage, SEPIA should be considered for sensations of heaviness or bearing down with or without actual prolapse, especially when accompanied by other keynotes such as nausea or irritability. (See Chapter 4.)

5. IGNATIA

A history of acute grief or disappointment with a picture of contradictory or "impossible" symptoms will usually point to IGNATIA. This pattern may occur at the time of miscarrying, as a complication obstructing the normal process, or suspected beforehand, as an authentic fear to be overcome. (See Chapter 6.)

6. SABINA

Tincture of the fresh, young branch tops, *Juniperus sabina*, N. O. Coniferae, the savin tree.

An important remedy for postpartum bleeding and indeed for functional uterine bleeding of all kinds, SABINA will be discussed again in Chapters 10 and 11. Often indicated for the prevention and treatment of miscarriage even when other more individualizing symptoms are lacking, it has a few general characteristics most suitably introduced at this point.

Also useful in the treatment of venereal warts and inflammations of the genitourinary tract in both sexes, SABINA corresponds mainly to conditions with excessive and painful uterine bleeding during or after miscarriage, childbirth, or menstruation. Typically intense and girdle-like, the pains often extend from sacrum to pubis, come in waves at regular intervals, and coincide with the passage of clots or tissue. At other times, the continuous background flow may intensify to the point of active gushing. SABINA is especially likely to benefit women who are full-bodied, of ruddy complexion, and excessively warm and intolerant of heat.

> *Case 8.2.* A single woman of 28 was five months
> pregnant with her second child when she came in for
> bleeding. At three months she noted some spotting with
> a recurrent Trichomonas infection but sought no
> treatment. By four months it was sufficient to require
> tampons to control it, but still she neglected to tell
> anyone about it. She consulted me only when it resumed
> a month later, being then comparable to a light period.
> The blood was dark, with big clots, cramping pain in her
> back and hips whenever she passed them, and some

mucus in her stools as well. She had had gonorrhea once with an IUD in place, and was powerfully built, weighing nearly 200 pounds and visibly uncomfortable in the heat. Recommending bed rest and SABINA 200 four times daily to control the bleeding, I sent her for an ultrasound, which confirmed the diagnosis of placenta previa. Within 48 hours she expelled a stillborn fetus of about 22 weeks' gestation, again alone and unattended, and required no further treatment.

SABINA should also be considered for ongoing vaginal bleeding and other typical complaints that have never resolved since a miscarriage at some point in the past, for prevention of miscarriage on the strength of such a history, or if miscarriage is imminent or threatening and other more distinctive symptoms are lacking.

7. CHINA

Tincture of dried bark, *Cinchona officinalis*, N. O. Rubiaceae, Peruvian cinchona or quinine bark.

Another leading remedy for postpartum bleeding and for ailments from bleeding, dehydration, and excessive loss of body fluids generally, CHINA will be discussed further in Chapters 10 and 11. The acute syndrome calling for CHINA is much the same as would be expected from excessive loss of blood, with chilliness, thirst, faintness, and a generalized shock-like state characterized by low or absent blood pressure, rapid and thready pulse, and the like. The chronic pattern is one of extreme and prolonged fatigue in the wake of such an episode.

> *Case 8.3.* A woman of 32 gave birth to her fourth child at home with no trouble, but was pregnant again within four months. A preliminary serology was positive, and her past history included two miscarriages and an abortion, but more detailed tests ruled out active or latent syphilis. At eight weeks, after an episode of cramping and bleeding that flooded through two pads but ended without passing any tissue, she no longer felt or tested pregnant. She consulted me two weeks later, after continuing to feel

143

excessively tired, weak, and chilled since the miscarriage. Her exam was entirely normal. CHINA 30 was suggested four times daily, and within a few days she was able to resume nursing and her other duties.

Abortion

The remedies to be considered for pain, bleeding, infection, or emotional problems following abortion or D&C are the same as for miscarriage, with the addition of two others:

1. CALENDULA

The great remedy for lacerations and abrasions of the skin and mucous membranes, CALENDULA can be equally healing to the uterine lining after an abortion or D&C (aptly known as a "scraping"), when it can be expected to feel raw, sensitive, or lacerated. In such cases, CALENDULA 30 may be given orally every few hours, and a dilute solution of aqueous CALENDULA Ø in sterile water or saline may be used for irrigation of traumatized tissues, four times daily or more often as needed for comfort.

2. PYROGENIUM

The sovereign remedy for early or threatening uterine infection following childbirth, PYROGENIUM will be discussed in Chapter 11. It may be used to prevent infection following an abortion when the lochia turns foul or rotten, or if fever or chills develop. In more advanced cases, emergency hospitalization and conventional treatment will be needed as well.

Nausea and Vomiting

Often dismissed as a simple hormone imbalance, this most common of all first-trimester complaints warrants further investigation. The progesterone surge of early pregnancy is approximated each month during the premenstrual or luteal phase, but persistent nausea and vomiting are unusual in the nonpregnant state. Nor can the chorionic hormones of pregnancy account for the fact that many healthy pregnant women experience no nausea or vomiting whatsoever.

Nausea and vomiting may represent simple biological tension between the instincts of procreation and self-preservation that every pregnant woman must somehow reconcile. To sustain a healthy pregnancy, the mother's immune system must learn to tolerate this single exception to its most basic programming, its instinct to locate, destroy, and expel all foreign elements. Indeed, to receive the advancing columns of embryonic tissue, the pregnant uterus must continually digest itself until placentation is complete by the end of the third month.

Even if the pregnancy was intended, planned, and hoped for, the surrender of physiological autonomy and personal liberty required to sustain it could naturally arouse considerable resistance on the most primitive biological and psychic levels. Nausea and vomiting may simply represent the most common symptomatic expression of a developmental process that normally takes weeks or months to accomplish and undoubtedly carries into extrauterine life as well. It is no small miracle that women are so well endowed with whatever it takes to make these adaptations as quickly and efficiently as they do.[3]

Although often amenable to successful treatment with remedies, the typical nausea and vomiting of early pregnancy can be expected to recur one or more times in the first three months or even after that, and the remedy may need to be repeated or changed more often than is customary in other acute situations.

1. SEPIA

With its underlying archetype of bioenergetic ambivalence at all levels, SEPIA is the remedy most often helpful for ordinary nausea and vomiting of pregnancy. It can sometimes be recognized in the character of the nausea itself, when intensified by the smell or thought of the foods usually preferred. A similar ambivalence may also be noticeable as a pointed dislike of friends, loved ones, and perhaps of the pregnancy as well that can seem exaggerated or out of character even to the patient herself, whether or not she manages to conceal it. Commonly regarded as irritable, "emotional," and selfish because of their need to be alone, quiet, and free of external responsibilities, SEPIA patients may expect to be cared for without having to ask.

Physical exercise is impossible in many cases, with the nausea aggravated by even a minimal effort such as getting out of bed or walking to the toilet, or by riding as a passenger in a car, boat, or plane. Equally noteworthy are the aggravation from not eating, and the almost immediate relief from eating a cracker or small bit of food, both typical of "morning sickness." All of these symptoms give the impression of a confused, ambivalent immune system groping for a middle path between the extremes of total merging with or outright rejection and expulsion of the pregnancy as a "foreign" substance.

SEPIA patients also commonly exhibit intolerance of fatty foods and the characteristic bearing-down pain or discomfort in the uterus, rectum, or bladder (or analogous sensations of sagging or heaviness elsewhere).

When indicated, SEPIA 12 or 30 may be given three times daily or more often for several days consecutively until better, and then resumed weekly as needed. With SEPIA 200, try three doses in 24 hours, repeating weekly if necessary and using SEPIA 12 or 30 as needed in between.

> Case 8.4. A married woman of 32 was nearly six months along in her second pregnancy when she was referred to me for recurrent nausea. Her typical morning sickness had resolved months ago without remedies but had come back recently when her two-year-old son began waking every night and coming into bed with them. Her husband amiably indulged this behavior, since his business allowed him to stay home and make up lost sleep during the day. Indeed, because he rarely helped with the child care or approved of her disciplinary efforts in general, his mere presence in the house regularly infuriated her at this juncture. The nausea was aggravated by eating too much or missing a meal and by walking or driving. SEPIA 200 was all the medicine she needed. After three doses in 24 hours, she completed the pregnancy without further incident, worked out a

more sensible division of labor with her husband, and had an easy home birth with his active support and encouragement.

2. PULSATILLA

Another superb remedy for nausea in pregnancy, PULSATILLA will usually be suggested by its characteristically mutable physical and emotional style and typical keynote symptoms like intolerance of warm rooms, improvement in the open air, and sensitivity to overeating, fat or rich foods, bread, milk, or fruit. (See Chapter 4.)

> *Case* 8.5. After a beautiful home birth and an abortion just five months later, a woman of 28 decided to try again and came in at about nine weeks with severe nausea, which she had not had in her earlier pregnancies. Although intensified by the smell of greasy foods or tobacco, it was still quite spotty, coming and going for brief periods during the day and night, and could usually be relieved somewhat by taking a stroll in the fresh air. I suggested PULSATILLA 200, three doses in 24 hours, along with the 6X tablets as needed throughout the day, and she was back to normal within a week, completing the remainder of the pregnancy and the birth without any difficulty.

3. NUX VOMICA

The pattern of symptoms calling for this remedy suggests nervous hyperstimulation, usually with typical keynotes such as drug abuse or intolerance, constipation or other autonomic dysfunction, and insomnia or ailments from lack of sleep or emotional excitement. (See Chapter 6.)

> *Case* 8.6. Eight weeks into her first pregnancy, a 35-year-old woman became intensely nauseated after drinking beer and then more or less continuously since catching cold a few days later. Her senses also seemed hyperacute, and even familiar smells such as car fumes

and cigarette smoke were amplified to the point of bringing on headaches. Even her usual cravings for alcohol, coffee, tobacco, and marijuana could no longer be indulged without immediate and disastrous results. NUX VOMICA 200, three doses in 24 hours, and 6X tablets as needed, were wonderfully calming to her nervous system. Her nausea quickly subsided, and she finished out the pregnancy without serious problems, giving birth at home as planned.

4. IGNATIA

As always, the indications for this remedy are to be found in a context of acute grief, sorrow, or disappointment, typically associated with "impossible" or contradictory symptoms and other evidence of nervous excitement, such as insomnia, trembling, drug sensitivity, and the like. (See Chapter 6.)

Case 8.7. A girl of eighteen was nine weeks pregnant when she came in complaining of nausea, headaches, and other seemingly unrelated complaints that followed soon after a breakup with her boy friend, who had gone off with someone else. Although the pregnancy itself was seen by her peers as a desperate attempt to be with him still, for the past six months she had planned to break off the relationship, leaving it to him to destroy the love that was still so dear to her. The nausea itself was very persistent and often accompanied by stabbing headaches, numbness of the hands, and episodes of blurred vision when letters and other objects appeared alternately larger and smaller than their actual size. Although these symptoms were greatly intensified by alcohol, coffee, and tobacco, she continued to smoke two packs of cigarettes daily. IGNATIA 1M, three doses in 24 hours, seemed to do the trick. After a week of hysterics, with head-banging and fantasies of murder and suicide, she finished her first year of college with good grades, giving birth to twins over spring break without serious difficulties.

5. PHOSPHORUS

Always to be considered for ailments of pregnancy, PHOSPHORUS is especially helpful for complaints arising from or heightened by an overactive imagination with exaggerated fears and a tendency to somatization. Other typical keynotes (burning pains, thirst for cold drinks, etc.) should also be looked for. (See Chapter 7.)

> *Case 8.8.* Six weeks into her first pregnancy, a 27-year-old woman came in for her first prenatal visit wide-eyed, excited, and already quite nauseated and light-headed on waking, when she had to force herself to eat but felt much better once she did. An art teacher in junior high school, she was happily married and delighted to be pregnant but so impressionable that she had had a migraine from visualizing herself with a Down's syndrome child. She was unusually thirsty for cold water and fruit juice and rather prone to stomach aches shortly after meals. After a round of PHOSPHORUS 200, she felt much better within a week and had a successful home birth seven months later.

6. NATRUM MUR.

Easily missed in the welter of early pregnancy symptoms, the NATRUM MUR. picture is most striking in its background tones of grief, sorrow, or disappointment and a resulting flavor of grimness and rigidity that defeats hope of improvement or change. (See Chapter 7.)

> *Case 8.9.* A woman of 36 was seven weeks pregnant with her second child when she consulted me for nausea, which was aggravated by coffee, alcohol, and tobacco, from waiting too long to eat, and from riding in the car. Both she and her husband seemed truly happy and excited about the pregnancy, as was their five-year-old son. Her main desires were for hot, spicy foods and warm tea and soup. NUX VOMICA 30 helped for a short time; but her marked improvement at the beach and unusual craving for salt reminded me that she had

149

almost left her husband three years ago, when he gave her a case of gonorrhea, and had taken him back only after considerable pleading and solemn oaths of love and fealty. In less than a week after one round of NATRUM MUR. 1M, her symptoms were nearly gone, and the remainder of the pregnancy and the birth followed without incident.

7. COCCULUS

Tincture of the powdered seeds, *Cocculus indicus*, N. O. Menispermaceae, the Indian cockle.

Still used by South Indian fishermen to stun their catch, this plant contains the alkaloid picrotoxin, which produces excitement and convulsions of the central nervous system. Homeopathically, the remedy has a special affinity for the vestibular organ of the inner ear and two other characteristic features that make it useful in the treatment of headache, nausea, and other nervous disorders with vertigo or dysequilibrium.

The first is a marked aggravation of all symptoms from riding in cars, boats, trains, and planes, which makes COCCULUS the leading remedy for simple motion sickness when other specific indications are lacking. Like SEPIA and a few others, it is also very sensitive to the smell or the thought of food, as are so many women in the early months.

The second is an equally strong sensitivity to loss of sleep, rivalling even NUX VOMICA in this respect, which is often coupled with a tendency to insomnia from emotional excitement, especially from the ongoing strain of nursing or caring for a friend or loved one who is chronically ill and the obsessive worrying that commonly results.

> *Case 8.10.* A woman of 23 was six weeks pregnant with her second child when she was referred to me because of severe nausea. Although normally hungry and largely free of symptoms for most of the day, she became intensely nauseated at the smell of food cooking and also while eating it, once it reached her stomach. She was also much troubled with headaches and motion

sickness, both of which had bothered her a lot as a child. COCCULUS 200 was speedily effective: her nausea was gone within 48 hours, her other symptoms also receded, and she sailed through the rest of the pregnancy and the birth without any major problems.

8. COLCHICUM

Tincture of the bulb gathered in springtime, *Colchicum autumnale*, N. O. Melanthaceae (Liliaceae), the meadow saffron.

Justly renowned as the source of colchicine, the great anti-gout principle, the meadow saffron is most often used homeopathically for the treatment of arthritic and rheumatic complaints that are aggravated by motion. Indeed, COLCHICUM rivals BRY-ONIA in its intolerance of walking, turning the head, or the slightest movement or activity of any kind, which applies not only to particular symptoms (joint pains, headache, nausea, etc.) but to the patient as a whole.

An equally general feature of COLCHICUM patients is their marked intolerance of smells (food, tobacco, diapers, car exhaust, perfume, etc.). Those likely to benefit from this remedy will usually be found lying or sitting quite motionless and as far away as possible from strong odors of any kind. There is also a tendency to bowel irritation with mucous or jelly-like diarrhea and a marked chilliness with sensitivity to cold or damp weather.

> *Case 8.11.* A woman of 21 was eight weeks pregnant with her first child and extremely nauseated. A hostess at a fancy restaurant, she complained that "I smell everything," from the hot sauce two tables away to the flowers across the room, every odor making her sicker. Her energy was also very inconsistent, particularly at work: when nauseated, she felt worse just from her usual duty of escorting guests to their table and seemed comfortable only when resting or lying still. Otherwise she seemed in good health and happy with her mate, although they were not yet married and hadn't intended to get pregnant quite so soon. With the help of COLCHICUM 30, she was much better within a

week: more energetic, less sensitive to smells, and able to work and eat with only minor discomfort. She had a healthy pregnancy and a lovely home birth without serious difficulty.

9. IPECAC

Tincture and trituration of the dried root, *Cephaelis ipecacuanha*, N. O. Rubiaceae, ipecac.

In emergency medicine, this South American plant is most commonly used to induce vomiting after accidental or deliberate ingestion of poison or drug overdose. In homeopathy the ailments for which IPECAC is most likely to be helpful are characterized by severe and constant nausea unrelieved by vomiting. It is therefore especially useful in the most severe or advanced cases, in which the patient is unable to eat and may require hospitalization and maintenance with IV fluids. It may also be helpful when there are no specific indications for other remedies or when other seemingly well-indicated remedies have proved ineffective. In such cases, profuse salivation is often a guiding symptom.

When these features are present, IPECAC can also be useful in the treatment of asthma, bronchitis, and the bronchiolitis of young infants. Along with SABINA and CHINA, it is often cited in the literature for postpartum bleeding as well.

> *Case 8.12.* Eight weeks pregnant with her second child, a woman of 32 was awakened in the night by severe epigastric pain and nausea that had been with her ever since. For two weeks she had retched and vomited from almost any food and remained nauseated for hours afterward, while the pain itself, which came and went without reason or pattern, seemed to gnaw at her stomach as if she were ravenously hungry. A registered nurse, she felt newly repelled and disgusted by the blood and gore surrounding her work ever since her mother's death in the early weeks of the pregnancy. Yet an occasional cigarette actually settled her stomach, and marijuana did so even more effectively. One week after

IGNATIA 30, she was much less nauseated and free of pain but still weak and unable to eat much more than warm milk and potatoes, retching whenever she felt hungry, after the smallest portion of food or drink, and from the least motion. IPECAC 30 was speedily effective in this difficult situation, and she was soon able to eat normally again, although she had other problems later in the pregnancy and the child was born with serious congenital anomalies.

10. SYMPHORICARPUS

Tincture of fresh, ripe berries, *Symphoricarpus racemosus*, N. O. Caprifoliaceae, the snow-berry.

This remedy is recommended in the literature for the most advanced or desperate patients with deathly nausea and paroxysmal or intractable vomiting sufficiently violent to produce blood. It merits a trial in stubborn cases that fail to respond to other remedies or when more specific or individualizing features are lacking.

Anemia and Malnutrition

Proper diet and nutrition in pregnancy comprise a vast subject with few universally valid rules and ample room for creative individual adaptation. It is helpful for patients to make a list of everything consumed in the course of a week to make sure that all major nutrients and food groups are well represented and tolerated. Ideally this should be done as early as possible but may be postponed for a while if nausea is a problem.

Insofar as possible, the diet should consist of fresh, unprocessed, whole foods to which as little as possible has been added and from which as little as possible subtracted. It is seldom necessary to prescribe specific diets or vitamin and mineral supplements other than for illness or hardship or unless the extra demands or stresses of career or work lead the woman herself to request them. Common sense suggests a few simple rules of thumb within which most people can figure out a daily caloric intake and total weight gain that makes sense for them.

A few simple "dos" and "don'ts:"

1. Try to eat often enough that the stomach is neither ravenously empty nor uncomfortably full.

2. Eat and drink regularly without relying on snacks or fast foods.

3. Eat when hungry, and eat foods that are appealing.

4. Plan meals for a week at a time to make sure that all major nutrients and food groups are well represented. Use a reference book listing the concentration of major nutrients in various common foods.[4]

5. Keep weight gain below 40 to 45 pounds. Larger amounts tend to make labor more difficult and uncomfortable, are harder to get rid of afterwards, and often create additional health problems besides.

6. Get professional help if appetite or weight gain is inadequate or excessive; if the food eaten is not properly digested or assimilated; or if a specially restricted diet (macrobiotic, vegan, yeast-free, etc.) is indicated for any reason.

Although still debated back and forth, adequate protein intake is important for the health of both mother and baby and may become clinically relevant later in pregnancy if edema, hypertension, and proteinuria suggest actual deficiency. The subject is thoroughly discussed in Brewer and Brewer[5] and will be reconsidered in Chapter 9. A simple vegetarian diet supplemented by dairy and occasional fish or fowl is perfectly adequate for most people.

The additional metabolic demands of pregnancy call for increases in the cardiac output and circulating blood volume of up to 30 or 40%. On the other hand, the blood itself may be noticeably thinner, the hematocrit or red-cell fraction often dropping to 34 or 35%, a level that would be considered anemic at any other time. The diagnosis of anemia in pregnancy is probably not justified unless the hematocrit reaches 32 or lower or perhaps 33 to 34 with symptoms such as fatigue, shortness of breath, or palpitations.

The two commonest types of nutritional anemia are readily differentiated by a complete blood count (CBC), which includes measurement of the actual size and hemoglobin concentration of the red cells. Iron-deficiency anemia is typically associated with red cells that are smaller and less concentrated than normal and appear pale and "washed-out" in the peripheral smear. By contrast, the anemia of Vitamin B_{12} and folic acid deficiency is characterized by red cells that are abnormally large and highly pigmented.

Iron-deficiency anemia is common enough that many obstetricians advocate routine iron supplementation throughout pregnancy. On the other hand, because all medicinal substances have the power to produce symptoms as well as cure them,[6] minerals taken in large doses for months at a time can perpetuate the same deficiency states for which they were originally prescribed.

In my experience, it is not at all uncommon for patients to remain or become anemic and exhausted after prolonged iron therapy or to improve when the iron supplements are discontinued. By far the best medicine for iron-deficiency anemia is prevention through diet, using a simple regimen such as the following:

1. Four times a week, eat foods naturally rich in iron.[7]

2. Four times a week, eat foods containing manganese,[8] an important trace element that facilitates absorption and assimilation of iron from the diet.

3. Avoid drinking coffee or tea, which can inhibit iron absorption from the diet.

4. If iron deficiency develops, chelated iron supplements (ferrous fumarate, ferrous gluconate) may be given for a month or two without serious difficulty.

In the healthy state, Vitamin B_{12} and folic acid are supplied by the intestinal bacteria. Usually seen in combination, *anemia traceable to B_{12} and folic acid deficiencies* suggests a disruption or change in the normal flora, itself often attributable to

a. radical dietary change, such as semi-starvation from severe nausea of pregnancy, excessive fasting, or unduly strict or prolonged adherence to "cleansing" or allegedly "mucus-free" diets; or

b. chronic or recurrent digestive problems, especially when associated with overuse of antibiotics and overgrowth of yeast or other less friendly species.

Under these circumstances, feeding B_{12} and folic acid supplements may not help until the normal flora is re-established with the aid of yogurt or *Lactobacillus* cultures if necessary.

My experience with calcium exactly parallels what has just been said of iron. Calcium is very plentiful and widely distributed throughout the food chain.[9] Large doses of calcium supplements are seldom required for more than a few weeks at a time and will often produce symptoms if continued for longer periods. Many women with leg cramps in early pregnancy report excellent results after taking calcium supplements for a short time but are bothered again in the later months if the extra calcium is continued and relieved only when it is stopped.

A simple and effective regimen for milk-drinkers and non-milk-drinkers alike is as follows:

1. Every day, eat a regular portion of one or more foods rich in calcium.[10]

2. Four times a week, eat one or more foods containing silicon,[11] an important trace element that facilitates the absorption and assimilation of dietary calcium.

Feeding the trace elements manganese and silicon to pregnant women in lieu of heavy iron and calcium loading was first suggested in the 1940's by the French physicist Louis Kervran, who claimed to have demonstrated *nuclear* or interatomic conversions between iron and manganese and similarly between calcium and silicon inside the animal body.[12] Although Kervran's hypothesis never received much attention or credence from the biomedical world, the dietary guidelines based on it have proven wonderfully effective in my experience.

Exercise and Regimen

Pregnancy, labor, and nursing are mighty athletic events requiring considerable physical and mental strength and endurance and best prepared for by a regular program of training and exercise.

Pregnant women have no opponents: their only reason for exercising is simply to *feel good*, to develop and use and take pleasure in their bodies as both instrument and purpose of all that is happening within.

A suitable exercise program for pregnancy should include the following elements:

1. Whatever exercise is chosen should feel good at the time and help keep the body fit. An aerobic component may be added if desired.

2. Exercise should be stopped well before the point of exhaustion and any time it doesn't "feel right."

3. Even when it is highly recommended or has always felt good in the past, the body signals when a given movement is no longer suitable or when it's time to quit. These signals should be listened to attentively and with respect.

Swimming is a superlative exercise for many pregnant women, because it develops stamina, endurance, and breath control as well as muscle strength, and the buoyancy of the water supports the added weight of the baby without excessive stretching, jarring, or tensing. Others who run daily—in some cases up to the day of delivery and again the day afterwards—have also had perfectly good and in some cases remarkably fast and easy labors. One woman in her late thirties told me that she felt perfectly well *without* exercising, and had no intention of starting just on *my* say-so. She too delivered beautifully.

What is true of iron and calcium applies even more directly to the use of drugs, including alcohol, coffee, and tobacco, and medications, whether pharmaceutical, herbal, or homeopathic. By definition, all medicinal agents have the power to go both ways, to cause symptom-alterations no less than to cure them, and the longer they are taken and the larger the dose, the greater the risk of trouble. Conversely, drugs or medications to which pregnant women are already addicted should be withdrawn gradually and only as their general health permits.

Meditation, prayer, and psychotherapy may be useful when a demanding career, stressful home life, or other personal problems or physical or mental symptoms make the pregnancy unpleasant or intolerable. Regular spiritual practice is also valuable under normal or healthy circumstances as an inner source of tranquility, guidance, and self-awareness.

Cystitis

Commonly felt in the first trimester and again in the final weeks, simple urinary frequency and urgency can result from the gravitational force of the pregnancy against the pressure-sensitive bladder mucosa and often requires no treatment. Actual urinary tract infections, on the other hand, with or without kidney involvement, can occur at any time and generally warrant professional help.

1. PULSATILLA

A superb remedy for reflex bladder irritation, PULSATILLA is wonderfully effective for many cases of simple frequency and urgency aggravated by warm, stuffy rooms, overeating or indulgence in rich or fatty foods, or emotional upset or excitement. Other typical PULSATILLA features will also be present. (See Chapter 4.)

2. SEPIA

Conditions relieved by SEPIA tend to be attributable to varying degrees of cystocoele, i.e., sagging or actual prolapse of the bladder into the vaginal vault, with typical symptoms of bearing down or incontinence, emotional irritability, and improvement from exercise. (See Chapter 4.)

3. STAPHYSAGRIA

Perhaps the classic remedy for "honeymoon cystitis," STAPHYSAGRIA is especially useful in cases of bladder involvement traceable to increased sexual activity, incomplete healing from a surgical procedure in the past, or passionate emotions such as anger, humiliation, or unrequited love that have been "swallowed" without being fully or adequately expressed. (See Chapter 6.)

4. CANTHARIS

Tincture or trituration of living insects, *Cantharis vesicator*, N. O. Coleoptera, the Spanish fly.

A tincture of this insect produces severe blistering on contact with the skin, and CANTHARIS in homeopathic dilution is a leading remedy for the treatment of second-degree burns and severe forms of bullous or vesicular dermatitis associated with blisters of varying size. CANTHARIS can also produce or relieve severe irritation or inflammation of the urinary passages and is usually the first remedy to be thought of for the treatment of acute hemorrhagic cystitis if other more distinctive symptoms are lacking.

Patients most likely to benefit from this remedy are tormented by constant urging and tenesmus with burning pain in the bladder and urethra both during and after voiding. CANTHARIS likewise inflames the male and female genitalia and enjoys an undeserved reputation as an aphrodisiac on account of its power to elicit intense and sometimes voluptuous sensations akin to those of sexual arousal. Unfortunately, like everything else connected with this remedy, such sensations are almost always painful and incompatible with normal function.

Emotional Problems

While no more or less common than at other times, emotional problems are rather more likely to surface and demand attention during pregnancy. Considerations of decorum or civility may well be swept aside by the insistent demands of growth, differentiation, and adaptation and the irresistible process that must somehow unite and reconcile them. Pregnancy is thus also an opportunity for personal growth, and the appearance of symptoms may provide a further impetus for necessary changes to be made. Homeopathic remedies have helped many pregnant women facing difficult choices to overcome the fear and pain that often stand in the way.

1. CIMICIFUGA

This remedy is often suggested by a picture of moroseness, dejection, negativism, or deep fears of insanity arising from a frightful experience with an earlier pregnancy or childbirth, miscarriage, abortion, or menstruation. The prescription is further corroborated by evidence of fragmentation or dissociation in the physical symptoms, such as headaches, neuralgia, or rheumatism that alternate or change abruptly, with uterine dysfunction either present or past. (See Chapter 3.)

Case 8.13. A 37-year-old woman was 15 weeks pregnant when she consulted me because of severe anxiety. Her first pregnancy had miscarried at six weeks. This time she was haunted by the memory that her mother had been four months pregnant with her when her sister was killed in a car accident, for which her mother had always held her responsible. No matter how often she heard the baby's heartbeat, a bit of spotting or a minor headache sufficed to revive her worst fears. After a round of CIMICIFUGA 200, the bleeding stopped, and she felt much calmer, although still convinced that "it will all be taken away in the end." At 24 weeks, soon after CIMICIFUGA 10M, she felt the baby kicking inside her and pronounced her womb officially "safe" for motherhood. The CIMICIFUGA 200 was repeated at 37 weeks, and CIMICIFUGA 10M at 42 weeks, when she finally went into labor and gave birth normally.

2. PULSATILLA

The emotions of PULSATILLA patients are almost too easy and appropriate, too readily accommodating or responsive to the demands of others, and often at the expense of self-assertiveness or self-esteem. Their obvious warmth and sincerity are so endearing that they themselves, no less than those closest to them, are easily beguiled into the path of least resistance and distracted from tougher issues of personal integrity. Other typical PULSATILLA keynotes and physical symptoms will ordinarily be present. (See Chapter 4.)

Case 8.14. A woman of 32 was 12 weeks pregnant with her third child when she consulted me for depression.

Although she did not want another child, she refused to have an abortion and took herself off antidepressants after a long history of dependence on them. She arrived in a truly pitiable state, dissolved in tears, prostrate from nausea and dizziness, and unable to get out of bed most of the time, let alone keep house or care for her children. Only at night with her family asleep was she free to pace or weep without fear of her husband, who was reluctant to accept the fact of her illness or incapacity. Nauseated after every meal, she could eat only tiny portions throughout the day, vomited milk and fatty foods, felt dizzy indoors, and had to open windows or go outside for relief. After PULSATILLA 10M, although still anxious about the pregnancy and tearful whenever she spoke about it, she could eat again more or less normally, her spirits revived, and she was able to get along better with her husband. After four weekly doses of PULSATILLA 200, she felt more energetic and able to do housework for the first time. One final dose of PULSATILLA 1M was given at 24 weeks, and she gave birth five months later without needing anything further.

3. SEPIA

Almost the opposite of PULSATILLA in this respect, the SEPIA patient tends to separate or detach herself from her loved ones and their demands and obligations, which are usually perceived as threats to her personal integrity. The presenting complaint may be a loss of affection for the spouse or older child or perhaps an ambivalence about the pregnancy itself, often accompanied by characteristic physical symptoms (nausea, sagging or heaviness) and relieved by taking time for herself and by vigorous exercise.

Case 8.15. Just six weeks pregnant with her fifth child, a woman of 34 was already nauseated "day and night," exhausted, and in a "foul" mood most of the time. After SEPIA 30, she was much less nauseated and able to nurse her youngest again, but the noise of her other children fighting made her yell and scream and break down in tears at the endless prospect of still more mothering on the horizon. SEPIA 200 was effective but had to be repeated several times, and other symptoms annoyed her until the end, as if in protest against the life of obligation and self-sacrifice that had become her lot.

4. IGNATIA

The picture of this remedy is dominated by repressed grief, sorrow, or disappointment, often betraying itself through emotional outbursts that seem inappropriate or out of character, or physical symptoms that are contradictory or anatomically "impossible." (See Chapter 6.)

Case 8.16. Thirty-two weeks pregnant with her first child, a 23-year-old woman came down with fever, a sore throat that kept her from swallowing, and a cough that made it easier to swallow, although she refused all nourishment except hot garlic and onion broth. No less improbable was her story: alcoholic at fourteen, when her father died, smoking marijuana daily at seventeen, a nervous breakdown at nineteen, married at twenty and living in an ashram. A year later, when her mother died, she left the ashram and got pregnant almost immediately. Her husband talked her out of an abortion but came home one night reeking from the smell of alcohol, now utterly abhorrent to her. Although saying nothing at the time, she awoke the next morning with the sore throat just described. When I saw her, she retched violently from the cough and was severely nauseated by the taste of her own cigarettes, yet could not or would not give them up. After a few doses of IGNATIA 200, her sore throat disappeared as rapidly as it had come, and she had a successful home birth soon after, although her marriage did not long survive it.

5. NUX VOMICA

The emotional picture of this remedy is pretty much what would be expected from a sympathetic nervous system under constant stress and therefore obliged to run on "emergency power" most of the time. Often "wired" or "keyed up" as if from amphetamines, NUX VOMICA patients may be irritable, aggressive, or "uptight," with little tolerance for others of differing persuasion or style. Most often the presenting complaint has to do with physical symptoms of imbalance in the autonomic or vegetative functions like eating, digesting, defecating, sleeping, or relaxing. (See Chapter 6.)

> *Case 8.17.* Six weeks pregnant with her second child, a woman of 25 consulted me for "nervousness" and shaking all over. Although she had abused amphetamines for nine years and shot coke and dilaudid a few times before she knew she was pregnant, she had been trying to stay "clean" since then and seemed genuinely to want the baby. After being nauseated for a few weeks, she was bothered mainly by nervous symptoms such as hysterical crying, irritable and impulsive behavior (yelling, slamming doors, breaking things), and "scatterbrained" or forgetful episodes. Because she continued to smoke pot and drink alcohol regularly and refused to count them as "drugs," I declined to help with a home birth, but she did very well on weekly doses of NUX VOMICA 200 and phoned some months later to thank me. They had a natural birth in the hospital, which also went off smoothly.

6. STAPHYSAGRIA

Patients needing this remedy usually have a history of having failed to recover properly after surgery, of having been abused, insulted, or humiliated, or of having experienced anger, disappointed love, or other emotions that were never fully expressed or worked through in the past. (See Chapter 6.)

7. ARSENICUM ALBUM

These patients often complain primarily of physical symptoms such as fatigue, chilliness, burning pains, etc. But even when they cannot define or articulate it, the underlying apprehensiveness and insecurity so characteristic of this remedy is seldom far away. Whether driven by anguish and restlessness or the need for order and detail, they usually look for health professionals willing to perform whatever tests or services it takes to reassure them. (See Chapter 7.)

> *Case 8.18.* A woman of 34 was 14 weeks pregnant with her second child, still quite nauseated at the thought of food, but above all apprehensive, consumed with worry about the pregnancy and other major changes in her life. Soon after beginning a doctoral program, she was panicked about buying a house, her husband's equally definitive career change, the new baby, and how she could possibly manage it all. After her first child was born by C-section, she was determined above all to wrest control of her next birth from the tyranny of the medical system. Yet she shied away from saying anything positive about the pregnancy, lest the envy or jealousy of her friends somehow undermine it. Equally fearful that the baby might be too large or too small, she often confused her fear of eating too much with her disgust at having to eat anything at all. After a round of ARSENICUM ALBUM 1M, she was able to complete the pregnancy in a more relaxed frame of mind and gave birth naturally at a birth center nearby. Within a year she was pregnant again, successfully completing her exams in her eighth month.

8. PHOSPHORUS

The PHOSPHORUS state involves empathic or even telepathic over-identification with the problems and sufferings of others, often to the point of taking on their symptoms or failing to distinguish the solidity of their own experience from the chimeras of their always fertile imagination. Confirmatory physical symptoms such as burning pains, cough, hoarseness, or thirst will usually be present. (See Chapter 7.)

9. NATRUM MUR

Whatever the illness, NATRUM MUR. patients usually present a history of chronic unhappiness or sorrow that have become hardened into a pessimistic or fatalistic attitude and a grim determination to survive. The physical symptoms also tend to have an unyielding quality suggestive of rigidity at many levels of functioning. (See Chapter 7.)

Case 8.19. In the sixth month of her first pregnancy a woman of 22 consulted me for genital herpes, which had reappeared a few months before; but mostly she was troubled with financial and personal problems. Although her husband had never held a job for more than a few months at a time, and she had left him twice already, she was still devoted to him and to having his baby. Inured to poverty and struggle since childhood, she had no memory of happier or more carefree times and resented most of all the "materialistic values" of American life, having no choice but to accept whatever meager sustenance she could manage to wring from it. Physically depleted and barely able to keep up with her part-time job, she slept ten hours a night, was prone to minor virus infections, and whiled away her boredom with day-dreams of riding on horseback across the plains or living on the land, tending her garden and chopping her own wood. She did well on two rounds of NATRUM MUR. 200 a month apart, finishing out the pregnancy in good health with no more herpes, and giving birth without incident. She called some months later to thank me in person for the remedies and above all for the chance to be heard.

CHAPTER 9

Late Pregnancy

SECOND TRIMESTER

Once the pregnancy escapes the bony pelvis and begins to show externally, downward pressure on the vagina and bladder is greatly relieved, and further growth exerts upward pressure against the abdominal contents, the diaphragm, and the respiratory muscles of the chest wall. Changing anatomical relationships thus often lead to temporary shortness of breath, heartburn, and indigestion during the fourth and fifth months. But on the whole and in the absence of other complications, most pregnancies are apt to proceed quite smoothly during this period.

Vaginitis

The normal secretions of the vagina tend to be thicker and more plentiful as the pregnancy develops, and the vaginal mucosa may be unusually moist or juicy as well. More individual changes in the normal acidity or alkalinity may favor overgrowth of common micro-organisms such as yeast (Candida albicans), Trichomonas, Streptococcus, or Gardnerella.

It is seldom necessary to treat vaginal discharges that are not irritating or offensive. Routine treatment with antibiotics or suppositories is often counterproductive and may provoke deeper and more serious problems. If troublesome symptoms persist, or specific pathogens warrant, homeopathic remedies chosen in the usual way are wonderfully safe and effective most of the time.

1. CAULOPHYLLUM

This remedy can be associated with a profuse, irritating vaginitis or discharge, especially toward the end of pregnancy and in association with other typical features (uterine dysfunction, arthritis of small joints, nervous excitement). It should be considered if a persistent or troublesome discharge lacks clear indications or has failed to yield to other remedies, since its resolution after CAULOPHYLLUM may contribute to an easier labor as well. (See Chapter 3.)

2. PULSATILLA

An excellent remedy for vaginitis, PULSATILLA corresponds to catarrhal inflammation of all mucous membranes, typically with copious, bland discharges and the usual general indications and modalities. In some cases the inflammation may be itchy, smelly, or irritating. (See Chapter 4.)

> *Case 9.1.* Sixteen weeks pregnant with her second child, a woman of 30 consulted me for vaginitis, which she had had for eight months since the beginning of her sexual relationship with the man whose child she now bore. While not yet in love with him and wanting more time with her son, she was thankful for his love and devotion, however long they might last. Yellow-green and malodorous, the discharge was positive for Trichomonas, and the friction of her clothes caused itching and burning for which only airing in the sun provided any relief. She was also mildly anemic, constipated from milk, and prone to indigestion from overeating. Her discharge cleared up soon after PULSATILLA 1M, her energy improved, and she phoned after the labor to tell me that all had gone well.

3. SEPIA

Another important remedy for vaginitis, SEPIA corresponds to sensations of heaviness or dragging, aversion to or discomfort from making love, and a marked improvement from physical exercise. The vulva and vagina tend to feel raw or irritated, and may show actual ulcerations, while the discharge can be of any type. Other typical SEPIA elements will usually be present. (See Chapter 4.)

> *Case 9.2.* In the sixth month of her second pregnancy a 23-year-old woman came in for her regular prenatal visit with a profuse, odorless, messy, but non-irritating discharge. Although her therapist had mentioned some sexual problems with her husband, she would say only that he was very busy lately and seldom home, and that she often felt irritable, "emotional," and shaky, most of all after caffeine, and had to eat something every few hours to steady herself. Yet she had enough energy to keep up with her son, do yoga, and bicycle eight miles a day. After SEPIA 1M she reported a brief intensification of all symptoms followed by slow, steady improvement, and there were no further problems with the pregnancy, which ended with a successful home birth.

4. KREOSOTUM

Tincture of volatile oils, chiefly guaiacol and creosol, obtained from the distillation of beechwood tar, creosote.

Formerly used as a preservative in the smoking process, the creosote of beechwood tar protects meat and fish from spoiling and is used homeopathically for illnesses with signs and symptoms of putrefaction. It is an excellent remedy for an excoriating type of vaginitis with a foul or even bloody discharge that stings and burns the vulva and vagina, particularly during sexual excitement or contact.

5. NITRIC ACID

Tincture of nitric acid solution, HNO_3, nitric acid.

Another remedy for severe cases with burning, stinging, and a thin, foul, corrosive discharge, NITRIC ACID has a special affinity for orifices where skin and mucous membrane meet (mouth, vagina, rectum, urethra) and is typically associated with ulceration.

> *Case 9.3.* Twenty weeks pregnant with her fourth child, a woman of 35 came in for her prenatal visit with a yeast infection like many she had had in the past and duly confirmed by smear. With almost no discharge, she felt dry, itchy, and uncomfortable from any friction such as tight clothing or lovemaking; occasionally she also felt sharp, needle-like pains extending upwards through the vagina. Otherwise, apart from mild discomfort on urination, she seemed to be in good health, craving ham and milk as usual. After NITRIC ACID 200, the itching and irritation subsided and did not come back. When her time came, the baby slid out fast and easy, well before I got there.

5. SANICULA

Tincture of the mineral waters of the Sanicula spring, Ottawa, Illinois, Sanicula water containing NaCl, $MgCl_2$, $CaCl_2$, $Ca(HCO3)_2$, $NaHCO_3$, NaBr, NaI, $CaSO_4$, K_2SO_4, B, Fe, Li, Al, and Si.

A constitutional remedy with a broad range of action, SANICULA (or SANICULA AQUA) is sometimes used in the treatment of venereal warts and vaginal infections with discharges smelling like old cheese or spoiled fish.

Genital Herpes

The herpes virus presents a special problem because of the potential risk that the mother may pass it to the fetus *in utero* or to the newborn as it exits through the vagina. Although herpes infection is very common in pregnancy and quite rare in the newborn, it is very serious and sometimes fatal when intrauterine or vaginal transmission does occur. While the mother's first lesion is by far the most dangerous and previously infected pregnant women usually have antibodies in the amniotic fluid, even recurrent lesions have been implicated in some instances. To be on the safe side, most obstetricians still advocate elective Caesarean section for active lesions discovered within four to six weeks of the due date.

Although women with genital herpes in pregnancy will often benefit from homeopathic care, consultation with a physician or trained health professional is strongly recommended, and self-care for lesions appearing late in pregnancy should be combined with regular medical and laboratory examinations. Many suspected lesions are not confirmed by culture. In any case, if there are no active lesions and the parents are ready to take responsibility for the outcome, the final decision about a home birth rightfully belongs with the parents.

1. SEPIA

A leading remedy for herpes of the vulva, labia, and vagina, SEPIA will ordinarily be indicated by its typical general features but may also be tried when more precise indications are lacking. (See Chapter 4.)

2. PHOSPHORUS

The general features of the remedy (e.g. burning pains, thirst, fears, hypochondriasis, etc.) will usually be prominent, and a lot of reassurance will be required. (See Chapter 7.)

> Case 9.4. Ten weeks into her first pregnancy, a 29-year-old woman was very excited and in resplendent health but spooked about genital herpes. Though already a veteran of six lesions in her pubic hair, the most recent had been only two weeks earlier; and as her imagination raced ahead to possible future scenarios, her big, lustrous eyes stayed riveted on me for protection. She was happily married and had no other medical problems. After a round of PHOSPHORUS 200, everything went smoothly until about 35 weeks, when she reported two lesions less than a week apart, both less prominent and severe than usual, but worrisome enough. After a Pap smear and several cultures were negative, I gave PHOSPHORUS

1M, and we decided to go ahead with the home birth, which went off beautifully and without a hitch.

3. NATRUM MUR.

As always, the general indications will be decisive in choosing this remedy: unending grief, a grim determination to survive, and concomitant signs of physiological rigidity or immobilization. (See Chapter 7.)

4. MERCURIUS

Trituration of metallic mercury, *Mercurius vivus*, Hg, quicksilver.

The great anti-syphilitic drug of Hahnemann's time, MER-CURIUS is important in the treatment of destructive or ulcerating lesions anywhere in the body, and of foul, slimy, debilitating excretions or discharges from any orifice. In the mouth, where mercury amalgam fillings may actually contribute to the problem, indications for the remedy include excessive salivation, foul breath, painful or abscessed teeth, diseased gums, and herpetic or aphthous ulcers. In the vulva and vagina, it may be useful for herpes or other infections with ulceration or offensive discharge. Also a leading remedy for dysentery, MERCURIUS should be considered for patients with bone pains, night sweats, or unwholesome discharges from any source whose symptoms are intensified during the hours of night.

5. THUJA

Tincture of fresh green twigs, *Thuja occidentalis*, N. O. Coniferae, the *arbor vitae* or tree of life.

Identified with another of the great chronic disease styles recognized by Hahnemann,[1] THUJA is indicated for patients whose symptom-picture is dominated by excessive growth or proliferation of tissue (warts, moles, cysts, tumors, hyperplasia) or a history of gonorrhea or other infections of the genitalia suppressed but not cured by conventional treatment.

> *Case 9.5.* Early in her first pregnancy, a 32-year-old woman came for her initial visit worried mostly about genital herpes. Most of her ten previous lesions had

been on the vulva, the latest only two weeks ago. In addition she had had numerous warts on her hands and knees as a child, all of them frozen off with liquid nitrogen, as well as a Bartholin çyst that had been drained surgically a few years back and several Pap smears that were positive for cervical dysplasia. Although in excellent general health, she had suffered from insomnia for many years and seemed very reserved and even secretive about her personal life. After THUJA 200 she had no lesions for several months, despite typical premonitory symptoms on two occasions, which had never happened before. At 32 weeks she developed an atypical lesion that was cultured twice but proved negative. Repeating the THUJA 200, we opted for the home birth, which went off beautifully.

Digestive and Bowel Complaints

Almost unavoidable in pregnancy, increased pressure on the rectum and congestion in the pelvis generally may well aggravate any tendency to constipation and also to hemorrhoids in the later months. Heartburn and indigestion are especially common in the second trimester, when the upward growth of the fetus begins to crowd the major digestive organs. Although many patients choose to live with minor complaints that pose no threat to the pregnancy, homeopathic remedies properly used have a great deal to offer them, and cannot harm.

Pre-existing colitis, ileitis, or inflammatory bowel disease may also flare up or recede during pregnancy, and are also amenable to homeopathic treatment, but require professional supervision, which takes us well beyond the limitations of this book.

1. PULSATILLA

An excellent remedy for heartburn and simple indigestion from overeating, PULSATILLA is effective for many patients who can no longer tolerate their usual meal, are forced to eat small amounts more frequently, and are sensitive to fat and rich foods, meat, bread, milk, or fruit and raw foods in particular. Like other symptoms of this remedy, the heartburn and indigestion may be especially prominent when the patient lies down for bed or tries to relax or sit still, and will usually be relieved by "keeping busy" or taking a breath of fresh air. Other typical features will also be present. Under these circumstances, PULSATILLA can be an excellent remedy for constipation as well. (See Chapter 4.)

> *Case 9.6.* Twenty-three weeks pregnant with her first child, a 29-year-old woman complained of heartburn after eating a banana or avocado. Since she was in good health otherwise and symptom-free as long as she stayed active, no treatment was given. At her next visit a month later, she was very uncomfortable in the heat, suffered a good deal from heartburn in the evening, and felt soreness of the left hip and sacroiliac, likewise relieved by moving around. Unable to eat her usual dinner, she would often burst into tears for no reason and wanted to be stroked and petted like a child. PULSATILLA 30 was superbly effective in this typical case: her symptoms gradually melted away, and the rest of the pregnancy and the birth proceeded smoothly.

2. SEPIA

Also frequently indicated for constipation, heartburn, and other digestive complaints, SEPIA is prescribed on the basis of its great themes: sagging muscles, heaviness or dragging-down sensations in the pelvis and rectum, emotional irritability and disaffection from loved ones, and marked improvement from physical exercise. With or without nausea, which may linger from the earlier months, the symptoms tend to be aggravated by movement or riding in a car, by the smell or thought of food, and above all by neglecting to eat. (See Chapter 4.)

> *Case 9.7.* A woman of 36 was 25 weeks pregnant with her third child when she consulted me for fatigue and heartburn after meals, no matter what she ate, which was even worse from not eating and often forced her to lie down. Her other complaints included bulging

varicosities on the labia, abdominal cramps after love-making, and an uneasy feeling that the baby would fall out whenever she stood up. Under these circumstances, she did not appreciate being reminded that infertility and the longing for more children had prompted her to see me many months before. Her sole relief came from yoga, which she taught professionally. After SEPIA 200 she developed hemorrhoids, which did not bother her; her indigestion quickly subsided; and she coasted through the later months and the birth without further difficulties.

3. NUX VOMICA

A splendid remedy for indigestion, gas pains, and constipation, NUX VOMICA is useful for ailments traceable to overindulgence in rich or spicy foods, stimulants, drugs, or medications, or to a "high-powered" or stressful lifestyle (long hours, demanding job, lack of sleep, nervous tension, irritability, etc.). Even when not obviously constipated or in pain from rectal spasm or a hard stool, NUX VOMICA patients usually benefit greatly from a good night's sleep and a normal bowel movement. (See Chapter 6.)

4. COLOCYNTHIS

Along with MAG. PHOS., this remedy is indicated mostly for abdominal pains of a cramping or spasmodic type, relieved by heat and especially by hard pressure such as bending double. The pains of COLOCYNTHIS are often precipitated by overt or suppressed anger and may be associated with irritable bowel syndrome in the form of diarrhea and blood or mucus in the stools. (See Chapter 6.)

5. STAPHYSAGRIA

Complementary to COLOCYNTHIS and often indicated after COLOCYNTHIS has acted, STAPHYSAGRIA corresponds to ailments after surgery or from suppressed anger and is useful for digestive system complaints such as colicky pain and inflammatory bowel disease. (See Chapter 6.)

175

6. CARBO VEG.

Indicated mainly for poorly oxygenated states of the blood, CARBO VEG. inhibits putrefaction of the foodstuffs by anaerobic bacteria in the intestine and promotes healthy assimilation and elimination through rebalancing the intestinal flora. Indigestion calling for CARBO VEG. typically presents as uncomfortable, gassy distention after eating that is relieved by passing gas in either direction, often with considerable force. The most likely culprit is a large meal, full of rich, heavy sauces, desserts, or other indigestible items unfortunately highly prized by the patient. There may also be evidence of impaired oxygenation elsewhere, with sluggishness, cyanosis, air hunger, and improvement from cold air or fanning.

7. SULPHUR

Whether for heartburn or gas, constipation or diarrhea, patients needing SULPHUR are generally overheated and intolerant of heat,and will exhibit other typical features, such as itchy eruptions, intolerance of bathing, thirst, cravings, extroverted style, and the like. (See Chapter 7.)

8. LYCOPODIUM

Another important digestive remedy, LYCOPODIUM has as much gassy distention as CARBO VEG. and also resembles PULSATILLA in its intolerance of overeating. Apart from its peculiar keynotes (right-sided symptoms, 4 to 8 P.M. aggravation, etc.), a useful indication can be an underlying fear of failure or incapacity, often unseen but never far away. (See Chapter 7.)

> *Case 9.8.* A 30-year-old woman was 28 weeks pregnant with her third child when she came for her prenatal exam complaining of severe indigestion, not necessarily after eating but always from 4 P.M. on. Not quite nauseous and difficult to describe, the sensation was "disgusting," almost painful, and caused her to sip milk all day long. More noteworthy than the symptom itself was her extreme reticence amounting almost to secrecy about her

feelings or the details of her inner life. For her second birth, she did not take our prenatal classes and did not want my nurse to come to the birth, which was rapid and easy like the first. Her prenatal visits were also infrequent to the point that she would not have come this time but for the indigestion, which thus seemed more worrisome to her than she cared or knew how to talk about. With little else to go on, I gave LYCOPODIUM 30X as needed, and she sailed through the rest of the pregnancy and the birth as before, with an outer serenity and enigmatic smile that now seemed more brittle and interesting but never divulged its precious truth.

9. ARSENICUM ALBUM

One of the great remedies for dysentery and food poisoning, ARSENICUM has nausea and vomiting as well as diarrhea, with the characteristic chilliness, exhaustion, restlessness, anxiety, burning pains, and thirst, all relieved by heat and aggravated by being alone. (See Chapter 7.)

> *Case 9.9.* A woman of 36 was 13 weeks pregnant with her second child and acutely ill with gastroenteritis. Visibly chilly and restless, she was tormented with cramps, stabbing pains, and spurts of diarrhea that sometimes escaped *en route* to the toilet and left her even more chilly and shaky afterwards. Worst of all were the retching and vomiting, which negated her extreme thirst and made it impossible for her to eat or drink anything. After a few doses of ARSENICUM ALBUM 1M, she was able to keep simple food and water down and made a rapid recovery, culminating in a home birth seven months later.

10. MERCURIUS

Another splendid remedy for dysentery, MERCURIUS corresponds to a foul or slimy diarrhea with mucus or blood, excessive saliva-tion, offensive sweat, and a tendency for all symptoms to be aggravated during the nighttime hours. It is also excellent for the nocturnal heartburn so commonly seen in pregnancy. (See Chapter 8.)

11. ROBINIA

Tincture of fresh bark of roots or young twigs, *Robinia pseudo-acacia*, N.O. Leguminosae, false acacia.

The major keynote of this remedy is gastric hyperacidity or dyspepsia, particularly from lying down at night, effectively preventing sleep.

> *Case 9.10.* A woman of 29 was six months pregnant
> with her second child when she consulted me for
> heartburn, mainly when lying down at night, which
> obliged her to take antacids to get to sleep. She was
> otherwise in good health. ROBINIA 30X as needed
> helped her through this nuisance in a very short time,
> and she had a second home birth without any difficulty.

Pelvic Pain

From the stitching pain of an early *corpus luteum* cyst to the Braxton-Hicks contractions of the later months, occasional abnormal or painful sensations in the pelvis are common in pregnancy and usually require no treatment. Homeopathic self-care is useful for persistent uterine or ovarian pain without diagnosable pathology requiring acute medical or surgical intervention. Accompanied by severe pain and fever in most cases, acute pelvic infections can easily endanger the pregnancy, and may warrant hospitalization even when appropriate remedies seem well indicated.

1. MAGNESIA PHOS.

The major indication for this remedy is severe, typically cramp-like pain in the uterus or ovary, causing the patient to double over and relieved mostly by heat. (See Chapter 6.)

2. COLOCYNTHIS

As with MAG. PHOS., the pains of this remedy tend to be crampy and relieved somewhat by heat, but firm pressure is usually most effective. Often there is a background of anger or indignation as well. (See Chapter 6.)

> *Case 9.11.* Soon after moving to the area, a 17-year-old woman was 22 weeks into her first pregnancy when she came in complaining of severe pain in the right groin. Although the pregnancy had been unplanned, both she and her boyfriend wanted to marry, seemed genuinely happy about the baby, and in any case had ruled out abortion for moral reasons. The pain, which had begun within a few days of their arrival, felt "like a muscle tightening," was made worse by standing or walking, lying on her back, or rolling over in bed, and was relieved mainly by sitting up and applying hard pressure with her elbow. She attributed it to the stress of trying to find an apartment, which she took very much to heart, "like a personal insult." COLOCYNTH. 200 was speedily effective. She remained in good health thereafter, giving birth at home with no trouble whatsoever.

3. STAPHYSAGRIA

This remedy corresponds to uterine, ovarian, or pelvic pain following unusual or excessive sexual activity, suppressed anger or humiliation, or a major surgical procedure. (See Chapter 6.)

4. LYCOPODIUM

This remedy will usually be prescribed on the basis of typical indications such as right ovarian pain, aggravated by overeating and at 4 to 8 P.M., relieved by passing gas, and accompanied by the characteristic anxiety. (See Chapter 7.)

5. LACHESIS

LACHESIS is useful for left-sided pelvic or ovarian pain that is most intense during or after sleep or from touch or tight clothing, and is relieved by a discharge of some kind. (See Chapter 7.)

6. LILIUM TIGRINUM

Tincture of fresh stalk, leaves, and flowers, *Lilium tigrinum*, N.O. Liliaceae, the tiger lily.

Useful in many female complaints, LILIUM TIGRINUM is associated with dragging, pulling, or bearing-down sensations in the pelvis; brownish vaginal discharges; and vehement or passionate emotional outbursts, with inner restlessness, hurried thoughts and movements, and improbable or exaggerated responses generally. For example, odd heart pains "like a hand squeezing and letting go" have been described radiating down the *right* arm and wandering about or alternating with other symptoms. LILIUM patients are typically overheated, subject to sudden flushes of heat, intolerant of warm rooms, and generally improved in the fresh air.

It has strong points of comparison with PULSATILLA, which is also excitable and intolerant of heat; SEPIA, with its intense bearing-down pains; and IGNATIA, which is even wilder and more outlandish. But its closest analogue is PLATINA.

> *Case 9.12.* After a brief relationship with a boy in his late teens, a woman of 23 found herself pregnant with his child. Both excited and terrified, she went to an abortion clinic but backed out at the last minute. Now living with him and committed to having the child, she came for her first prenatal visit at 14 weeks with a history of passing dark brown blood for ten days and severe drawing-down pains in both groins that often forced her to lie down. Unusually nervous and apprehensive as a result, she felt excessively hurried in her thoughts and movements and driven to try to do everything at once. After a round of LILIUM TIGRINUM 200, the pain and bleeding stopped, and she finally settled into the pregnancy, which she completed without further difficulty, giving birth at home with her new husband in devoted attendance.

> *Case 9.13.* A woman of 29 was visiting from another town and only six weeks pregnant when she came in for intermittent vaginal bleeding and a feeling of pressure or bearing down low in the pelvis that felt as if her organs

were falling out. For the past year she had had similar symptoms of lesser intensity after her menstrual periods, while seven years before that her first child had been stillborn. Her vital signs were stable, but the pelvic exam revealed an enlarged, tender left ovary and a foul-smelling discharge with the color and texture of chocolate pudding, which cultured out *Bacteroides* and other anaerobic species. After three or four doses of LILIUM TIGRINUM 200, the pain and bleeding promptly subsided, and she finished out the pregnancy in good health, phoning me after the birth to report that everything had gone well.

7. PALLADIUM

Trituration of the metal, Palladium, Pd.

This remedy has a strong affinity for the right ovary, for pains relieved by pressure or rubbing, and is associated with ailments from wounded pride, coupled with excessive need for approval. PLATINA is complementary.

8. PLATINA

Trituration of the metal, Platinum, Pt.

Widely used in the chemotherapy of ovarian cancer, metallic platinum is employed homeopathically for ovarian pains and complaints, particularly on the left side, and when associated with bearing-down sensations and intensified during or after sexual intercourse. The external genitalia may be exquisitely hyper-sensitive to touch, either to the point of heightened sexual arousal or in some cases precluding it altogether.

In the mental sphere, patients needing PLATINA may seem unduly proud or haughty or quietly cultivate an idealized or perfected vision of themselves or their abilities, even or perhaps especially when their actual personal fortunes have suffered. In a typical somatization, external objects or people may literally be "seen" as smaller or farther away than they really are. Finally, the symptoms tend to alternate with one another, making a strange and vivid picture.

LILIUM TIGRINUM and PALLADIUM are complementary.

Two Important Remedies
for Late Pregnancy

Two remedies are indicated for so many second- and third-trimester ailments that they could almost be thought of as constitutional remedies of late pregnancy itself. Although often prescribed in the early months as well, they are particularly relevant to maternal physiology once placental development is well established and should be thought of on the basis of their overall symptom-picture even more than for any specific complaints.

1. SULPHUR

A constitutional remedy *par excellence* for many types and phases of chronic illness, SULPHUR corresponds beautifully to the added metabolic demands of pregnancy, when pre-existing tendencies are often heightened and even well-established patterns may need to be modified or changed. Often traceable to increased heat production, SULPHUR complaints tend to be characterized by excessive intolerance of warm rooms, warm baths, warm clothing, or becoming warm in bed, and to manifest in a rough, crude, or uneven way, involving some areas or aspects much more strongly than others. Whatever their presenting complaint, most SULPHUR patients will also exhibit other typical features like burning pains, itching, and redness, all aggravated by heat and relieved by cold, with extreme thirst for cold drinks, ravenous hunger or faintness at 11 A.M., and cravings for sweets and alcohol. SULPHUR's late-pregnancy repertoire includes indigestion, vaginitis, hemorrhoids, edema, toxemia, dermatitis, and much else. (See Chapter 7.)

> *Case 9.14.* At sixteen weeks in her first pregnancy, a 31-year-old woman came in feeling "run down" and faint, particularly in the heat. With a history of periodontal disease and a major depression following her mother's death, she seemed remarkably ebullient and good-humored, engaging in rough banter with her husband and laughing uproariously at her own infirmities. Rather heavily built and slovenly in appearance, she ate

enormous meals with gusto, washed them down with large quantities of water and soda, and felt faint if she waited too long in between. Already a little edematous and water-logged, she was also awakened in the night by dryness and itching in the nose. After a round of SULPHUR 1M, her energy seemed more balanced, her appetite less extreme, and she finished the pregnancy in good shape, giving birth at home without difficulty.

Case 9.15. Early in her first pregnancy, a 33-year-old woman consulted me for a Class III Pap smear showing severe dysplasia, which reverted to normal after SEPIA, IGNATIA, and CALCAREA CARB. 200. She came back one last time at about 37 weeks, after antibiotics prescribed for a urinary tract infection had left her swollen and clumsy and given to irrational fears about her husband and baby. Most striking of all was her transformation from her customary cold-blooded state into feeling flushed and overheated most of the time, opening windows in the middle of winter, and drinking gallons of ice-cold soda water. SULPHUR 1M acted almost magically here, and she wrote soon after to report that she had given birth to a nine-pound son with no further problems.

2. KALI CARBONICUM

Trituration of the salt, potassium carbonate, K_2CO_3.

Easy to forget and often difficult to recognize, the picture of KALI CARB. tends to fit patients who seem crabby, vague, and evasive in telling their symptoms, as if somehow ashamed or reluctant to reveal themselves too fully. Yet, despite their sometimes humdrum character and unappealing presentation, the symptoms are usually sufficient to point to the remedy once it is thought of.

First, the remedy is full of nagging, stitching pains, "side aches," and lumbago, in which the painful areas often need to be pressed hard or rubbed for relief. Second, both the patient herself and most of her particular complaints tend to be aggravated in the wee hours of the morning, especially from 2 to 4 A.M., making KALI CARB. an important remedy for insomnia late in pregnancy. Whether awakening to urinate, from pain or anxiety, or with no other symptoms at all, the patient may be unable to get back to sleep, perhaps troubled by practical matters or vague doubts and fears that remain ill-defined. In a manner suggestive of ARSENICUM ALBUM, many patients needing KALI CARB. are tormented by diffuse or free-floating anxiety when awake, especially when alone or less distracted by the tasks of daily life.

Also resembling ARSENICUM ALBUM in its overall chilliness and sensitivity to cold, KALI CARB. is an excellent remedy for almost any ailment in late pregnancy dominated by neurasthenic features as described above. It has seen good service in the treatment of cough and catarrh, pneumonia or bronchitis, and in delayed or prolonged convalescence following any severe or debilitating illness, with chronic fatigue, anemia, or weight loss.

> *Case 9.16.* Six months into her second pregnancy, a woman of 30 came for her regular prenatal visit complaining of heartburn, insomnia, and sporadic flu-like feelings of weakness that would overtake her suddenly and force her to lie down for 30 minutes at a time. Most noticeable after eating too late in the evening, even tea and honey, the heartburn often woke her up at 3 A.M. But she also awoke at that hour on other nights, feeling chilled even under the covers, and worrying about how she would manage to care for the baby, not to mention their shaky finances, while most of the time she enjoyed her favorite meat or sausage dishes with impunity. All of these symptoms were narrated in a whining, monotonous style, as if calculated to bore the listener or prevent their being heard or integrated in a meaningful way. After a round of KALI CARB. 200, her sleep and energy improved, the other symptoms receded into the background, and she had a quick and easy home birth with no complications. When she developed hay fever in her next pregnancy, KALI CARB. once again saw good service.

Case 9.17. Late in her first pregnancy a woman of 24 caught cold and developed a sore throat and a cough that were worse on lying down and in the wee hours of the morning, when they would sometimes wake her. Her slow recovery from this illness had left her feeling weak, clammy, and mildly feverish, with leg cramps that roused her from sleep at 3 A.M. Her most worrisome complaint was a vague apprehension about the birth and a fear of "the unknown" that was difficult for her to define or even talk about. Within days after KALI CARB. 200, these residual symptoms vanished, and she went on to have a beautiful home birth with no problems.

THIRD TRIMESTER

Throughout the last three months, rapid growth and differentiation of fetal organs and tissues are accompanied by increases of up to 30% in the maternal blood volume and cardiac output, with some thinning of the blood, the hematocrit or red-cell fraction often dropping to 34 or 35%, while the blood pressure may rise to 140/90 in the final weeks, a level that would be considered hypertensive otherwise.

At the same time, both to accommodate fetal growth and to facilitate expulsion, the pubic symphysis and sacroiliac joints are widened and loosened, significantly increasing the pelvic dimensions, while the breasts continue to enlarge and develop. As the birth approaches, the baby drops back into the pelvis to assume its final position, relieving pressure on the diaphragm, ribs, and stomach but redirecting its full weight downward against the bladder, rectum, and lower extremities.

Although unavoidable to some extent on the basis of these changes and often further complicated by hereditary influences, many typical complaints of the last three months can be relieved more safely and effectively by homeopathic remedies than by any conventional means.

Arthritis, Neuralgia, and Rheumatic Complaints

1. CAULOPHYLLUM

This remedy is useful for pain and inflammation of the fingers and toes with the typical uterine dysfunction, muscular weakness, and nervous excitement or a past history of such. (See Chapter 3.)

2. CIMICIFUGA

Commonly associated with severe headaches and neuralgic pains, CIMICIFUGA also corresponds to diffuse or localized sensations of bruised soreness and arthritis or rheumatism of the larger joints. It will be indicated mainly by its other features: uterine dysfunction, mental and physical fragmentation and alternation of symptoms, choreiform movements, and the like. (See Chapter 3.)

3. PULSATILLA

An important arthritic remedy, PULSATILLA has pains that are typically mutable, wandering freely from place to place, and highly vulnerable to overheated or stuffy rooms, overeating and fatty or rich foods, and any emotional upset or excitement. (See Chapter 4.)

4. SEPIA

The remedy par excellence for loose joints and sagging muscles, SEPIA can do wonders for the sacroiliac and other aches and pains of late pregnancy that are directly related to the weight of the baby pressing down on the pelvis and lower extremities and are relieved by strenuous exercise. Other typical keynotes, such as bearing-down sensations, intolerance of fat, and irritability or loss of affection for loved ones, are also likely to be present. (See Chapter 4.)

5. ARNICA

Used mostly after acute trauma to the soft tissues, ARNICA is excellent for falls, sprains, or strains with bruising and may also be used as a liniment, applied directly to sore or injured muscles, joints, or ligaments, but never to an open wound. (See Chapter 5.)

6. NUX VOMICA

Superb for muscular tension attributable to loss of sleep, constipation, drug abuse, overstimulation, or simple nervousness, NUX VOMICA is often indicated for patients who work too hard, play too hard, and find it difficult to relax, with stiffness or tightness of neck, back, or limbs a common result. (See Chapter 6.)

7. BRYONIA

A major remedy for joints, tendons, ligaments, and bursae, BRYONIA corresponds to acute or subacute inflammation with pain that is exquisitely sensitive to the least motion and relieved by immobility or lying on the painful side. It is nearly specific for ordinary bursitis of the shoulder and for pleurisy or pleurodynia. Other BRYONIA features (thirst, gruffness, intolerance of sensory or mental stimulation) will also be present. (See Chapter 6.)

8. RHUS TOX.

The leading remedy for simple sprains, pulled or strained muscles or ligaments, tendinitis, lumbago, etc., RHUS TOX. has tight, pulling pains that accumulate at rest, become sharp on beginning to move, "limber up" from continued movement, and return as fatigue develops, requiring frequent changes of position. Most patients feel worse from exposure to cold or damp weather, and are relieved by hot drinks and by warmth in general. (See Chapter 6.)

> *Case 9.18.* Seven months pregnant with her first child, a 31-year-old woman came in tired, swollen, and incapacitated by a pinched nerve in her sacrum, which "locked" when she stood up and caused her legs to buckle from trying to support her weight. A dancer by training, she could prevent or mitigate the symptoms only by regular exercise and not becoming overtired. After a round of RHUS TOX. 200, the whole syndrome quickly faded into the background and never bothered her again. Remaining in good health thereafter, she had a lovely home birth with no complications.

9. MAGNESIA PHOS.

Primarily a neuralgic or antispasmodic remedy, MAG. PHOS. soothes the sharp, cramplike, shooting, or lancinating pains often seen with sciatica and typically relieved by pressure or rubbing but mostly by a heating pad, hot bath, hot water bottle, or the application of heat in any form. (See Chapter 6.)

> *Case 9.19.* Seven months pregnant with her second child, a 29-year-old woman was greatly troubled by stabbing pain in the left shoulder, "like a knitting needle," and by sciatic pain down the back of the right leg, both relieved by heat and massage. Both were old complaints, the shoulder pain having started on the right side in the early part of the pregnancy and the sciatica originating at about the same time with her first baby. After a round of MAG. PHOS. 200, both pains subsided promptly, and she remained well, giving birth at home after an easy labor with no complications.

10. COLOCYNTHIS

Equally useful in sciatica, COLOCYNTHIS is used for pains like those of MAG. PHOS. but relieved chiefly by hard pressure, heat being rather less important. In many cases, a background of anger or indignation can be elicited. (See Chapter 6.)

11. COLCHICUM

Like BRYONIA, COLCHICUM corresponds to painful inflammations of joints and connective tissues that are aggravated by the least movement or activity and relieved by remaining as still as possible. The typical chilliness and sensitivity to odors and to cold, damp weather will usually differentiate it. (See Chapter 8.)

> *Case 9.20.* A 27-year-old woman was four months pregnant with her third child when she consulted me for backache, mainly in the lower back but extending into the thighs as well. Labor-like in its style and intensity, the pain would often stop her in her tracks

and force her to lie down and remain as motionless as possible. She also felt chilly, regardless of the temperature, and continued to have nausea off and on, mostly from odors such as the smell of food cooking. COLCHICUM 200 was very effective, and she wrote afterwards to report that the remainder of the pregnancy and the birth had gone well.

12. KALI CARBONICUM

This remedy comes in handy for nagging back and side aches that have to be rubbed hard for relief, may awaken the patient at 2 to 4 A.M., and are associated with a certain kind of diffuse complaining or querulousness that is difficult to appease or pin down.

> *Case 9.21.* A 28-year-old woman was seven months along in her first pregnancy when she developed stitching pains in her ribs that prevented her from sleeping on either side. A little worse after overeating and somewhat better from rubbing, they were not affected by heat or cold, and there was nothing else remarkable about them except that they often awakened her at 3 A.M. and interfered with her sleep. After KALI CARB. 200, her side aches promptly subsided, and she remained well thereafter, finishing the pregnancy with a lovely home birth.

13. LEDUM

Tincture of dried leaves and twigs at flowering, *Ledum palustre*, N. O. Ericaceae, marsh tea.

A good remedy for puncture wounds, LEDUM is widely used preventively after insect stings and animal bites. In more advanced cases with anaerobic infection developing in the wound, there may be bluish discoloration and a surface coldness to the touch, while the patient herself may require ice or ice-cold applications for relief. LEDUM has also been used effectively for the relief of arthritic and rheumatic complaints with similar characteristics.

14. RUTA

Tincture of whole, fresh plant, *Ruta graveolens*, N.O. Rutaceae, rue.

Used mostly for bone bruises and injuries to the periosteum like being kicked in the shins or hit squarely in the face or the back of the foot, RUTA is also helpful for bone pains of a similar type without actual injury, such as "shin splints" or periostitis elsewhere in the body.

Hemorrhoids

Essentially dilated veins of the rectal mucosa, hemorrhoids may be visible externally as bluish, grapelike swellings around the anal opening and can usually be felt protruding with or shortly after the bowel movement. Harmless and all but inevitable in late pregnancy if the familial influence is strong, they need not be treated unless they itch or hurt or show a tendency to bleed.

1. PULSATILLA

A great venous remedy, PULSATILLA is good for hemorrhoids in patients whose symptoms are highly mutable, with typical hot and cold phenomena, intolerance of warm rooms, overeating, or emotional excitement, and improvement in the fresh air. (See Chapter 4.)

2. SEPIA

With its well-known sensations of heaviness or sagging down, sometimes with an actual "ball" sensation in the rectum, SEPIA when indicated is splendid for hemorrhoids. Other typical symptoms, such as loss of affection for loved ones or the improvement from vigorous exercise, should also be present. (See Chapter 4.)

3. NUX VOMICA

With its late hours, nervous hyperstimulation, and indulgence in rich food and drugs, the NUX VOMICA lifestyle is very likely to put extra strain on the liver and hence the hemorrhoidal veins as well. NUX patients are prone to hemorrhoids, aggravated by constipation and lack of sleep, and often have difficulty curtailing the habits that do them harm. (See Chapter 6.)

4. SULPHUR

A sovereign remedy for late pregnancy in general, SULPHUR corresponds to patients in an overheated state from greatly increased blood volume, with congestive phenomena in the skin and elsewhere, including the rectum. It is accordingly helpful for hemorrhoids that are hot or burning, aggravated by the heat of the bed or after a bath, and accompanied by the typical thirst and intolerance of heat generally. (See Chapter 7.)

> *Case 9.22.* A woman of 30 was eight months pregnant with her second child when she came in for her prenatal visit complaining of rectal pain and discomfort from recurrent hemorrhoids. Often bothersome since giving birth to her first child in her native country, the hemorrhoids had gotten much worse this time since coming to the United States under difficult circumstances. After some improvement from PULSATILLA, they came back worse than before, with a searing pain after stool that continued to plague her all day long and throughout the night. She also felt overheated most of the time, even in the winter, and intolerant of heat in any form, feeling faint in the sun, consuming vast quantities of ice-cold liquids, and putting her feet out from under the covers on the chilliest nights. SULPHUR 200 was magically soothing to her rectum, and helped her to pull off a lovely home birth without any problems whatsoever.

5. LACHESIS

Full of bluish swellings and discolorations, LACHESIS is useful for hemorrhoids that are sensitive to touch, friction, or tight clothing and aggravated during or after sleep. (See Chapter 7.)

6. AESCULUS

Tincture of the ripe kernel, *Aesculus hippocastanum*, N. O. Sapindaceae, the horse chestnut.

The classic remedy for hemorrhoids in the absence of other guiding symptoms, AESCULUS is especially useful in more advanced cases with the characteristic sensation of needles sticking in the rectum. Otherwise, as with other remedies given on more or less routine or generic indications, it should be given low in a 6C or 12C and for a few days at a time, until a response occurs.

7. HAMAMELIS

Tincture of fresh bark from twigs and root, *Hamamelis virginica*, N. O. Hamamelidaceae, witch hazel.

Perhaps the greatest of the venous remedies in the absence of other indications, HAMAMELIS has no peer in the treatment of simple trauma or injury to the veins. Its rectal symptoms are primarily congestive, with sensations of swelling and soreness and bleeding of a passive, venous type. In general, it is closely related to ARNICA and PULSATILLA.

Varicosities

Like hemorrhoids, varicosities or dilated superficial veins of the lower extremities are familial and to some extent permanent once their elastic limit is exceeded. Although quite harmless, their considerable nuisance value includes unattractive swelling, discomfort, heaviness, and soreness, all amenable to homeopathic treatment. Usually found on the thigh or calf, they also occur on the vulva or inside the vagina. Phlebitis is uncommon and not dangerous unless the deep veins are also involved.

1. PULSATILLA

PULSATILLA is given on much the same general indications for varicose veins as for hemorrhoids. (See Chapter 4.)

2. SEPIA

As always, the hallmarks of SEPIA for varicose veins are the related symptoms of heaviness or bearing down in the pelvis and rectum with the typical syndrome of irritability or ambivalence toward loved ones and improvement from exercise. (See Chapter 4.)

3. CARBO VEG.

Seldom indicated for varices alone, CARBO VEG. indicates some degree of systemic deoxygenation, with diffuse cyanosis and other signs of deep-vein involvement (edema, stasis ulcers, coldness to touch, etc.), the typical need for cold air and fanning, gassy indigestion, and the general tendency to sluggish healing and prolonged convalescence. (See Chapter 6.)

4. LACHESIS

The chief indications for this great remedy would be any marked left-sidedness, constrictive sensations or sensitivity to touch or tight clothing, and the paradoxical aggravation from sleep, with improvement from being awake and about, seemingly in defiance of gravity. (See Chapter 7.)

5. HAMAMELIS

Much more for the "typical" case with rather vague or non-descript symptoms of congestion, heaviness, swelling, or soreness, HAMAMELIS is the best remedy to try if more distinctive indications for other remedies are lacking. In such cases, it should be given low (6C, 12C) and often.

Abnormal Presentation

It is rarely necessary or desirable to turn babies from the breech or transverse into the vertex position before 32 weeks or so, because at least half will convert spontaneously by then, with some chance of turning breech again. In the final weeks, as the ratio of amniotic fluid declines and the baby attains its greatest size, a successful version will be more likely to remain in position until delivery but also more difficult to achieve, especially after engagement has occurred.

These considerations leave a short time of maximum opportunity between 32 and 36 weeks for a first baby and perhaps somewhat longer for a second or third.

Converting a breech or transverse presentation with homeopathy illustrates both the elegance of the classical method and the mediocre results of trying to short-cut it. The literature is unanimous in recommending PULSATILLA for abnormal presentation, and my experience amply confirms that it will work about 40% of the time in a healthy woman lacking strong indications for other remedies. But the likelihood of success is even higher if the remedy clearly matches the totality of the symptoms.

> *Case 9.23.* Having had no prenatal care whatsoever, a woman of 30 was 33 weeks pregnant with her fourth child and in obvious distress, pacing the floor and sighing deeply, fanning herself as she walked, and relieving herself with loud, resonant belching. On examination, the baby was clearly breech. Of these three major problems, the most urgent seemed to be her illness, which she attributed to repeated episodes of bronchitis and pneumonia in the past, the drugs she had been given to subdue them, and a recent flare-up of indigestion from rich food and overeating. Within two days after a round of CARBO VEG. 200, she was greatly improved, and the baby had turned as well. At her next visit two weeks later, I agreed to do the home birth after all, and it too was successful, despite a postpartum fever that resolved in a few days and that CARBO VEG. would probably have helped to clear up sooner, if only I had thought of it.

If the patient is otherwise well, asymptomatic, and lacking clear indications for other remedies, PULSATILLA 30 may be given three times daily for several days, followed by the 200 and 1M at one-week intervals if necessary. If the baby remains breech after three weeks, it will probably be easier to deliver in that position and should therefore be left alone.

> *Case 9.24.* A 23-year-old woman had had an uneventful first pregnancy until she became slightly anemic at about 32 weeks and was placed on iron therapy for a month, with good results. At her 34-week visit, the baby was breech, and PULSATILLA 30 was given three times daily for three days, during which time she felt strong fetal movements and sharp pains low in the pelvis. When I examined her a week later, the baby had turned, and it remained vertex until the birth, which followed without a hitch a few weeks later.

Bleeding

Persistent vaginal bleeding in the last trimester is almost always a serious matter. "Bloody show" on the eve of labor can involve surprisingly large quantities of bright-red blood with little or no mucus but rarely lasts for more than a day at most. Contact bleeding from cervical polyps or cervicitis can occur after sexual intercourse but also subsides very quickly.

Both placenta previa and abruption or premature separation of the placenta, the principal causes of late bleeding, are dangerous to both mother and baby and often require hospitalization and emergency treatment. In most cases, homeopathic remedies will be unnecessary or insufficient; and those to be considered are the same as for postpartum bleeding. (See Chapter 10.)

Hypertension and Toxemia of Pregnancy

Once major causes of prematurity and maternal and infant death, the dreaded complications of hypertensive disease, proteinuria, and ultimately renal failure and convulsions have to a great extent preempted the schedule and format of modern prenatal care. Yet even now, lacking any unifying explanation, their pathogenesis remains mysterious, their treatment empirical, and their very definition inflated by fear. What follows is not a formal theory and certainly not a solution, but only a series of observations and a simple hypothesis to summarize and account for my own experience.

First, the blood pressure quite commonly rises as high as 140/90 mm. in the last three months, in response to the increased cardiac output and circulating blood volume of late pregnancy. Likewise, in proportion to the thinning of the blood, the kidneys readily allow more protein to escape into the urine, between "trace" and 1+ on the dipstick, a level often associated with mild to moderate swelling of the feet, hands, and face. Wholly consistent with a healthy pregnancy outcome, these common abnormalities in themselves seldom result in toxemia, and can safely be monitored and corrected with diet and homeopathic remedies if necessary.

The blood pressure is normally sensitive to moment-to-moment changes in posture, activity, nutritional status, and emotional factors, by no means the least of which can be the patient's fear of drastic medical intervention. For all of these reasons, I tend to give less weight to a single reading, or to how *high* the blood pressure can be made to go, than to its baseline level, or how *low* it will go if simply allowed to do so.

The best way to measure it would therefore be with the patient asleep or as completely relaxed as possible and unaware of being tested, a good clinical approximation being a few moments' rest with the patient lying on her left side (never on the back!). In most cases, this maneuver alone will lower both systolic and diastolic readings by 10 to 20 mm. each, thus demonstrating both an appropriate postural adaptation and good flexibility in the mechanism generally. If the recumbent reading is within the normal range, and there are no other danger signals (1+ protein or higher, excessive edema or weight gain, hyperactive reflexes), nothing further need be done at this point beyond frequent and careful monitoring.

My experience supports the Brewers' claim that dangerous levels of protein can often be prevented from escaping into the urine simply by eating a high-protein diet to maintain a high blood level. But even vegetarian patients rarely have to exceed their natural inclinations unless the dipstick gives a reading of 1+ or higher, and then for only as long as it remains out of range. In any case, for whatever reason, in thirteen years of a home birth practice encompassing over six hundred births, only one patient had to be hospitalized for toxemia, and she too gave birth vaginally at 38 weeks without complications or sequelae.

If significant hypertension and proteinuria develop in spite of a good diet and otherwise healthy pregnancy, homeopathic remedies may be tried, as long as the patient is monitored closely.

1. SULPHUR

An excellent remedy for pre-eclampsia, SULPHUR is helpful for patients with hypertension, edema, proteinuria, and other typical but exaggerated late-pregnancy complaints associated with excessive heat production, such as thirst, redness, and intolerance of heat. (See Chapter 7.)

Case 9.25. At 24 weeks a 38-year-old woman pregnant for the first time was found to have twins, the diagnosis confirmed by ultrasound. Otherwise in excellent health, she came in at 32 weeks energetic and in good spirits but with ankles and fingers swollen tight and her face flushed and puffy. The dipstick read 3+ for protein, and I could hear the blood pressure at 200 mm. even before I released the stopcock. Suspecting a reflex sensitivity to the cuff itself, which I have documented in a number of patients, I let off the pressure and pumped it up a second time, obtaining a new reading of 160/110. After three doses of SULPHUR 200, she reported a massive diuresis, and at her next visit a few days later, the swelling was much reduced, the protein 2+, and her blood pressure had fallen to 150/100, once more on the second try. After a few more doses of SULPHUR 200, the swelling was minimal and her energy and spirits were high, but her blood pressure never went below 150/100 or her proteinuria below 2+. In the end, I figured that these readings were probably normal for a woman of six feet weighing 200 pounds at this stage of pregnancy, and I decided to do nothing further than simply watch her closely. At 38 weeks she went into labor and had healthy six-pound twins at home after a slow labor with no problems afterwards.

2. APIS

Tincture of the venom, *Apis mellifica*, N. O. Insecta, the honey bee.

The familiar consequences of a bee-sting—stinging pains, localized swelling, redness, and heat—furnish a useful metaphor for the homeopathic employment of APIS in internal diseases, most notably in nephritis and toxemia. Its classic symptoms of oliguria, thirstlessness, and intolerance of heat correspond to a more severe or advanced degree of renal involvement than SULPHUR, a free and easy urination indicating that the remedy is acting favorably.

NATRUM MUR. is complementary.

Eclampsia with convulsions is a genuine emergency, potentially fatal for both mother and child, and warrants immediate hospitalization and medical intervention. I have never treated and would not attempt to treat such a case at my level of skill with homeopathic remedies alone.

CHAPTER 10

Labor and Childbirth

The intensive work of childbirth is ordinarily completed within a few hours and easily forgotten after months of gestation and the years of parenting to follow. Yet it remains the ultimate emotional and physical challenge that most pregnant women anticipate and prepare for, the biological moment of truth wherein all their hopes and fears for themselves and their children are concentrated and put to the test.

In a fast or easy labor, the successive stages often overlap or merge smoothly into one another, such that changes in breathing, vocalization, feeling-tone, and body language are adequate to monitor its progress without intrusive medical procedures. When the process is "stuck" or simply requires a longer time, definite stages are more accurately identified by physical examination and are correspondingly more useful clinically as well. I have therefore retained the concept of stages in the loose sense of milestones to be passed by each woman in her own time and in her own way, rather than as standards or expectations of performance or behavior.

THE INITIATION OF LABOR

Premature Labor

Although neither the ideal nor the actual length of pregnancy can ever be precisely known, the diagnosis of prematurity is warranted if labor begins or threatens at a time when the baby is less than fully developed or well before the predicted date, if the last period and measurements of fetal size are in agreement.

On the other hand, if active labor begins prematurely because the baby is seriously deformed or the placenta incapable of supporting further intrauterine life, artificial prolongation of the pregnancy is neither practical nor desirable. Because they can work only insofar as the individual patient is responsive to them, homeopathic remedies can help women in premature labor clarify for themselves whether the pregnancy is still viable or should be allowed to complete itself at that point.

The remedies useful in premature labor are more or less the same as for "false" labor, and in both cases their purpose is open-ended: 1) to help stop the labor if the pregnancy is still viable and the contractions signify only excessive uterine irritability; or 2) to help it proceed to completion if the baby is already dead or moribund, or has a better chance to survive outside the uterus.

1. CAULOPHYLLUM

As always, the prime indications for this remedy are, first, the typical uterine dysfunction, with weakness and nervous excitability; and second, if a similar syndrome appears imminent or threatening or has occurred in the past. Confirmatory signs such as neuralgias, rheumatism of the fingers and toes, or a profuse, irritating vaginitis, may also be present. (See Chapter 3.)

2. CIMICIFUGA

A leading remedy for prevention and treatment of premature labor in the absence of other indications, CIMICIFUGA is also useful in severe cases with established uterine dysfunction, mental and physical fragmentation or alternation, and disabling headaches, neuralgias, or arthritis. As with CAULOPHYLLUM, it can be used to treat premature labor or prevent it if it is imminent or threatening or has occurred in the past. (See Chapter 3.)

3. PULSATILLA

Always in the running for nearly every contingency, PULSATILLA will usually be suggested by its characteristic general features, such as changeable symptoms and emotions, circulatory instability and intolerance of warm rooms, restlessness, etc. (See Chapter 4.)

4. GELSEMIUM

An acute remedy with much the same flavor as CAULOPHYLLUM, GELSEMIUM features flu-like symptoms of weakness, trembling, aches and pains, chills, and emotional excitement along with a labor that stalls or "piddles" but still goes on. (See Chapter 5.)

"False" Labor

Meaningful only after the labor has actually stopped, the term "false" labor suggests an imitation of the real thing with more or less strong and regular contractions that may go on for many hours but do not progress or sustain themselves and are ineffective in dilating the cervix. Unlike premature labor, it occurs more or less at term with the baby fully viable, true labor following within a few days to a week at most. It could be thought of as a variant of dysfunctional labor that eventually stops altogether.

Most cases I can recall were in second or later pregnancies, when I would spend the night at the house to be on the safe side, and the morning would bring no more than the same sporadic contractions that had been happening for days or weeks already. Since many perfectly normal, healthy labors also begin in the same way, timely and well-chosen remedies can often indicate the shortest and safest way out of this dark forest as well.

Although a genuine nuisance for everyone, false labor seems to be a normal variant or even a kind of rehearsal that can actually shorten the rest of the labor when it finally gets in gear. In other cases, labor can progress normally for a time, stop completely for up to a day or so, and then take up essentially where it left off, also typically without ill effects for mother or baby.

The principal remedies to be considered are the same ones as for premature and dysfunctional labor. (See below.)

Late Onset and Postmaturity

Although such calculations are unavoidably imprecise, pregnancies that continue well past term deserve more careful attention. Postmaturity encompasses many of the same issues as prematurity and dysfunctional labor, and is also covered by some of the same remedies. As always, the effectiveness of homeopathic remedies in initiating labor depends on their detailed similarity and overall "fit" with the total symptom-picture of the patient.

Whether handed down by friends or relatives, or previously experienced or imagined by the patient herself, obsessive fears or "horror stories" about birth, labor, or parenting may prevent labor from starting or interfere with its progress at any point. Even in active labor, emotional issues can seriously interfere with, arrest, or actually reverse its progress, sometimes in defiance of well-established "scientific" principles.

> *Case 10.1.* In labor for the first time, a woman of 28 was already fully dilated when I got there, with the baby's head halfway down the vagina. Thinking only to applaud her achievement, I predicted that the baby would be born within the hour, but my words seemed to have the opposite effect of stopping her labor in its tracks. When I examined her, the cervix had reappeared and pulled the baby's head back up into the uterus, and no remedy I gave would persuade it to relax its hold. Although it took me a while to realize it, she needed more time to outgrow her subservient role in her husband's clannish family and gave birth easily in a few hours, once this important inner work had been accomplished.

When the pregnancy goes well past term, the baby must be monitored closely. Apart from the cumbersome "non-stress" test, which requires a fetal monitoring device, there is much to be learned from using an ordinary fetoscope for an hour or so every few days. With time and patience, it is a simple matter to detect or fail to detect normal variability of the heart rate spontaneously and in response to fetal movement. The most precious gift of the midwife, which no busy obstetrician or high-tech equipment can ever duplicate, is *herself*, her own undivided and loving attention.

1. CAULOPHYLLUM

The indications for this remedy are essentially identical to those already summarized under premature labor, with simple weakness of the female reproductive organs and a certain component of apprehension and nervous excitement, the classic CAULO-PHYLLUM syndrome. (See Chapter 3.)

2. CIMICIFUGA

Also to be considered in the absence of other more specific indications, CIMICIFUGA will often be suspected on account of a history of a frightening or unnerving experience of childbirth, miscarriage, or abortion in the past. The most important confirmatory evidence is provided by the usual dysfunctional uterine contractions with signs of alternation or mental and physical fragmentation in the present. (See Chapter 3.)

3. PULSATILLA

The indications for PULSATILLA are likewise identical to those for premature labor, including the characteristic pattern of emotional and physical mutability, restlessness, and a strong need for affection and emotional support, as well as the usual physical keynotes. (See Chapter 4.)

4. GELSEMIUM

For late onset or postmaturity, GELSEMIUM should be considered for trembling or "jitters" from the excitement of anticipating the birth, resembling "stage fright" and accompanied by the usual muscular weakness. (See Chapter 5.)

5. IGNATIA

Always to be considered when emotional factors seem predominant, IGNATIA may help patients who are unnerved by grief, sorrow, or disappointment and exhibit contradictory or anatomically "impossible" symptoms and other typical nervous phenomena. (See Chapter 6.)

Spontaneous Rupture of Membranes

In the home setting, leaking or gushing of amniotic fluid prior to labor is rarely a serious problem and can usually be managed successfully without antibiotics or any need to induce labor or rescue the baby by Caesarean section. Tears in the amniotic sac are common and usually repair themselves quickly, while the amniotic fluid is produced continuously, such that even major losses are replaced in a matter of hours.

For 24 to 48 hours following the leak, it is important to check the temperature, vital signs, fetal heart rate, and any vaginal secretions or discharges every four to six hours for evidence of bacterial infection. Most of the heavy police work is done by the friendly bacteria, which keep foreign species away efficiently and unobtrusively. Remedies are useful if the labor is difficult or complicated, or if infection occurs or threatens, as happens much more commonly in the antiseptic hospital environment, where unfriendly, antibiotic-resistant organisms are much more likely to flourish. In these latter cases, remedies alone may not be sufficient, and the ones to be considered are the same as for postpartum infection. (See Chapter 11.)

THE CONDUCT AND MANAGEMENT OF LABOR

The Stages of Labor

In actual practice, each labor is a unique experience that can get "stuck" at any point, and the same remedies may be needed throughout if indicated by the total symptom-picture. For purposes of study, however, the events of labor may be divided schematically into three more or less distinct "stages."

The *first stage* spans the interval during which the baby remains *in utero* and the cervix is gradually abolished by effacement and dilatation. It begins with the first sustained and progressive contractions and ends when the cervix is fully dilated and the widest diameter of the baby's head or presenting part enters the vagina. There may be a slight pause in the contractions at this point. Often there is a variable period of "back labor" in the first or early second stage, when the baby's head rotates anteriorly to clear the pubic arch.

The *second stage* corresponds to the descent of the baby down the vagina, beginning with the achievement of full dilatation and ending with the birth of the baby through the vaginal opening. Frequently the second-stage contractions are associated with a slower type of breathing, producing a deeper and more open sound, and culminating in the grunting and bellowing of the actual pushing. Many women feel no definite urge to push and should not be pressured or forced to do so. There is no fixed time limit for how long the baby can safely be allowed to remain in the vagina, as long as it is monitored closely and there are no indications of distress.

The *third stage* begins with the birth of the baby and ends with the delivery of the placenta.

Monitoring the Labor

Since foreign bacteria introduced into the vagina from the outside are likely sources of infection, the midwife and other birth assistants owe careful attention to personal cleanliness and hygiene. Thorough scrubbing of hands and nails with a surgical brush and mild soap is adequate for most home births, while hospital and clinic settings very properly require more elaborate aseptic and antiseptic procedures.

Whenever possible, frequent or unnecessary examinations should be avoided and simpler, gentler alternatives devised for finding out whatever needs to be known. One reason why home birth works so well is that being a guest in people's homes makes it inappropriate for the midwife or obstetrician to tell them how to give birth or how to live their lives.

In the home setting, the job description becomes simply to *be there* for the woman and her family, which I take to mean noticing as much, doing as little, and behaving as unobtrusively as possible. A vaginal exam or even a quick check with the fetoscope takes on new meaning if performed only when asked for, or for a definite reason deserving formal permission and perhaps a modicum of ceremony.

My goal is to earn the same privileges and duties as a trusted friend of the household, mostly by looking, listening, puttering around in the next room, washing the dishes, and paying attention to the "feel" of the experience as well as the technicalities of the labor. In this manner, it is usually possible to follow the progress of the labor very closely with a minimum of interference.

While not always easy to achieve in practice, a related and equally important priority is to encourage the other participants to take over as much of the actual work of managing the labor as they can. Even when needed mainly to bless the division of labor already agreed upon, the midwife can always play such eminently useful roles as identifying specific tasks to be performed and teaching and supervising basic skills as required.

Rediscovering one of life's core experiences through the medium of self-care makes home birth exciting and rewarding in a way that can never be forgotten. It is for these deeply human as well as practical reasons that emergency childbirth should be taught as part of the basic technical preparation for home birth. Indeed, some of my proudest memories are of births that happened before I got there, or in spite of my best efforts to control them.

THE FIRST STAGE

Failure to Dilate: Prolonged, Difficult, or Dysfunctional Labor

Although likewise vague and imprecise, these terms refer to common problems that most people can learn to recognize. Because each labor is unique, accurate judgment relies more on how the patient feels and functions by her own standards than on averages or external measures of performance. Technical procedures can then be used for further clarification, to diagnose specific obstacles or blocking influences, and to facilitate prognosis and management. I have somewhat arbitrarily assigned dysfunctional labor to the first stage, because it usually begins during effacement and dilatation, but the same principles are applicable later as well.

Any remedy may be useful at any stage of labor, and the total symptom-picture consistently yields better results than a prepared recipe. In those numerous cases where patterns develop and resolve too quickly to warrant detailed case analysis, the indicated remedy must be chosen on the basis of its well-known general features. As in earlier chapters, many other remedies have been omitted simply because I haven't used them often enough.

Finally, even well-selected remedies do not always work, and complications may persist until something else is done. In order to illustrate the distinctive features of the remedies, homeopaths like to present their best cases, omitting all the painful and tedious hours when the same ones were tried without effect. But let the reader beware of wishfully thinking that remedies alone can eliminate suffering, or of overlooking the obvious possibility that healing may simply fail to occur.

1. CAULOPHYLLUM

This remedy tends to work best early on, lacking more distinctive symptoms to indicate other remedies and before the dysfunctional pattern is so advanced and the woman so exhausted that other supportive measures (IV fluids, fruit ices, sleep) may be needed before any remedies will work.

Under these circumstances, CAULOPHYLLUM may be suspected whenever the uterus feels soft even at the height of the contraction, the labor stationary in its rhythmic progress, and the woman exhausted out of proportion to any objective evidence of useful work done. Usually short and unstable, the contractions may be feeble and infrequent or sharp and spasmodic, and are typically felt low in the pelvis rather than at the top of the uterus, where they would do the most good. Often there will be trembling, shaking, or other signs of nervous excitement as well. With these early warning signs, the remedy may be given right at the beginning, without requiring a vaginal exam to confirm them. (See Chapter 3.)

Case 10.2. After a hospital labor complicated by hypertension, an otherwise healthy woman of 31 came to see me for constitutional treatment before trying again, checking her own blood pressure anxiously and often. At the first visit, it was 150/90 mm. on my exam table but only 130/90 in the chair, her chin quivering nervously as I took it. With PULSATILLA and some reassurance, she was soon pregnant and remained healthy throughout, needing only a few remedies and a lot of attention. When she went into labor, she dawdled for hours, making very little progress until we gave her a dose of CAULO-PHYLLUM 200, whereupon she promptly switched into high gear and gave birth less than two hours later.

Case 10.3. After one hospital birth under general anesthesia and a second after premature labor at 30 weeks, a woman of 28 had a healthy and uneventful third pregnancy except for some bleeding and cramping in the last three months. She went into labor right on time but very desultorily at first, with weak contractions felt mostly low in the pelvis. With the help of CAULO-PHYLLUM 30, she went into active labor and gave birth in less than an hour, needing the remedy again for flabby contractions and bleeding afterwards. Her postpartum course was entirely normal.

Although most often thought of in the first stage because of failure to dilate, CAULOPHYLLUM can be equally helpful for uterine dysfunction complicating descent or expulsion or for problems with the placenta, after-pains, or postpartum bleeding.

2. CIMICIFUGA

While similar in type to those of CAULOPHYLLUM, the contractions of CIMICIFUGA tend to be more violent, and are apt to be accompanied by other disturbing symptoms as well. The patient may appear gloomy, dejected, or morose, with persistent doubts and fears about her ability to continue. In more advanced cases, fears of insanity or psychotic ideation and behavior may present an alarming picture. In addition, there will usually be evidence of fragmenting or dissociation on the physical level in the form of alternating symptoms, coarse involuntary movements or grimaces, or severe headaches or neuralgias that interrupt the continuity of the labor. (See Chapter 3.)

Case 10.4. After two abortions, a woman of 29 married and became pregnant again easily, opting for a home birth in part because of irrational fears of the hospital stimulated by films such as "One Flew over the Cuckoo's Nest." The pregnancy was healthy and uneventful, as was most of the labor, but she "lost it" briefly during transition, when the continuous pain revived her old fears of hospitalization. CIMICIFUGA 200 was instantly calming to her, and she gave birth soon after without further difficulty.

Case 10.5. After four years of marriage a woman of 21 had her IUD removed and got pregnant almost immediately. Although generally healthy, she had had a lot of cluster headaches in the past, as had her mother. Late in the pregnancy, tormented with nightmares and fears of losing her husband and baby, she told me that her mother had been depressed and under psychiatric care for a long time. She went into labor at term, soon after her membranes ruptured, but could not progress beyond 7 cm. A nagging backache responded well to KALI CARB., but her old fears and persistent negativity did not. CIMICIFUGA 200 was quickly effective in this situation, and she gave birth soon after. Her mental symptoms resurfaced after a breast infection six weeks postpartum, and once again she responded to CIMICIFUGA 200, followed by constitutional treatment with other remedies. Although more easily recognized when the contractions reach their peak rhythm and intensity, CIMICIFUGA may be needed and helpful at any stage. It is also an important remedy for retained placenta, after-pains, bleeding, and postpartum depression.

3. PULSATILLA

Useful at every stage of pregnancy and labor, PULSATILLA will usually be thought of because of the general symptoms such as emotional or vasomotor instability and marked improvement from drinking fluids, cool fresh air, and simple affection or caring. Although commonly indicated early in labor, it should not be overlooked for problems with expulsion, bleeding, or the placenta. (See Chapter 4.)

Case 10.6. After a healthy first pregnancy greatly benefited by SULPHUR 1M in its final months, a 30-year-old woman had a short, easy labor until the second stage, when the baby got "stuck" at a +1 station, her contractions stalled, and she became cross and weepy. After CHAMOMILLA 30 was given without obvious benefit, she asked for fresh air and some quiet time with her husband, which together with PULSATILLA 30 helped her push the baby out without further delay.

Case 10.7. After an uneventful second pregnancy and a long night of "false labor" the week before, a woman of 25 called me again in the wee hours, this time greeting me with twin daughters in her arms when I arrived. "You're a little late, Doc!" she teased, her high spirits charming away my embarrassment at not having diagnosed the twins to begin with. Her uterus remained hypotonic after the birth, and she continued to bleed rather heavily, feeling faint and chilly yet wanting the windows open for relief. PULSATILLA 30 was speedily effective in this typical situation: shreds of membrane and placental fragments were expelled, the bleeding slowed to a trickle, and her pulse and blood pressure reverted to normal levels. After that little scare, the rest of her postpartum course proceeded without difficulty.

4. SEPIA

Although more often indicated after labor than in the middle of it, this great remedy can relieve the characteristic heaviness and bearing-down pains whenever they occur if the symptoms agree. It is used chiefly for bleeding, retained placenta, prolapse, and other postpartum complaints. (See Chapter 4.)

5. ARNICA

Often given semi-routinely after the birth to prevent bruising and soreness, ARNICA should be considered if the baby is very large or the pushing long and difficult, if Pitocin is used for induction or augmentation, or when there are other reasons to suspect or anticipate trauma to the soft tissues. In such cases, the remedy may be given during the labor as well. (See Chapter 5.)

6. BELLADONNA

During the first stage of labor, BELLADONNA may be helpful for a rigid or swollen cervix that fails to dilate when other classic symptoms are present to indicate it, including sudden or violent onset, headache or other pains that are worse from jar, and dilated pupils or wild-eyed expression. A similar picture may occur after the birth, in cases of postpartum bleeding with violent gushing or spurting of hot arterial blood. (See Chapter 5.)

7. CHAMOMILLA

Extreme sensitivity to or intolerance of pain is the hallmark of CHAMOMILLA, whatever the condition. In labor, the patient is likely to be cross and irritable whenever the pain is intensely felt, demanding inordinate attention and support yet unable to accept or make use of them when offered. The bowels are often disordered as well, with loose stools, flatulence, or simple hypermotility. (See Chapter 5.)

> *Case 10.8.* After a successful home birth, a married woman of 25 became pregnant again and developed pleurisy in the eighth month, for which BRYONIA 30 was very effective. The labor was long and difficult and felt primarily in the back until KALI CARB. 200 helped the head to rotate anteriorly. In the second stage the pains became unendurable, and she began to scream like a fish-

wife, hurling violent imprecations at her husband, with whom she was perpetually quarreling, and also at me and anyone else who ventured too near. CHAMOMILLA 30 was quickly effective in this classic situation, and she gave birth easily without further trouble.

Case 10.9. After an uneventful first pregnancy, a 29-year-old woman was already in active labor when I got there, running short laps around her tiny living room and forbidding me to get close enough to examine her or to listen to the baby. She did want something for the pain, however, and I gave her a dose of CHAMOMILLA 30 whenever she slowed down long enough to take it. Without delay or fanfare or indeed any friends to help her, she gave birth in her bed with her pets in attendance, and only her thanks for it afterwards to suggest that the remedy had played any role.

8. GELSEMIUM

In labor, the indications are much the same as for CAULO-PHYLLUM: dysfunctional contractions with muscular weakness and exhaustion; trembling, shaking, or nervous excitement; and chills, joint pains, and muscle aches reminiscent of a flu-like illness. Often swollen and rigid, the cervix may fail to dilate or remain spasmodically closed.

GELSEMIUM should be considered when the symptoms indicate CAULOPHYLLUM but have progressed to an advanced stage, or when the latter remedy has been tried but fails to act. Although typically thirstless, GELSEMIUM patients generally feel better from urinating and should therefore be encouraged to drink and empty the bladder regularly. (See Chapter 5.)

9. NUX VOMICA

Often overlooked in favor of the typical "female" remedies, NUX VOMICA has come to the rescue in many instances where the labor is obstructed by a full bladder or rectum with painful and ineffectual urge to urinate or defecate owing to spasm of the corresponding sphincter muscle in the perineum or pelvic floor.

Even early in labor, the remedy should be thought of when the patient feels a strong but unproductive urge to go to the toilet with the contraction, especially if other NUX VOMICA elements are present, such as irritability, hyperstimulation, or craving for or intolerance of stimulants. If the bladder or rectum happens to be full, mechanical evacuation by catheter or enema may be necessary as well. (See Chapter 6.)

10. KALI CARBONICUM

In many normal labors, usually late in the first or early in the second stage, the fetal occiput must undergo back-to-front rotation, and further molding may be required for it to slip under the pubic arch. KALI CARB. is often indicated when the labor gets "stuck" at this point, and becomes difficult and tedious until the maneuver is accomplished. In other cases, anterior rotation never occurs, and the baby is born "sunny-side-up" in the occiput-posterior or OP position.

Either way, the result is apt to be "back labor" with the typical KALI CARB. indication, a nagging lower backache felt between and also during the contractions, which are likewise felt primarily in the back and relieved somewhat by vigorous rubbing or pressure. Such patients are apt to walk or sit with their hand held firmly against the lower back or will plead with their mate or attendant to apply the pressure for them. Other KALI CARB. characteristics, like the middle-of-the-night aggravation and nagging or complaining behavior, may also be noted. (See Chapter 9.)

> *Case 10.10.* When her first baby died of congestive heart failure at a few hours of life, a woman of 26 became pregnant again the following year and remained strong and healthy throughout, with a number of minor complaints. Throughout the first stage of labor the baby's head remained posterior, and dilatation was impeded by a persistent backache, for which her only relief was in begging her husband to press on it as long and hard as possible. Within minutes after a dose of KALI CARB. 200, the head rotated to the front, she achieved full dilatation, and the birth followed without further delay.

Case 10.11. After three hospital births marred by hallucinations from Trilene with her second and severe bleeding on Demerol after her third, a woman of 32 was determined to have her last birth at home. Although she had had no serious health problems during the pregnancy, the baby seemed consistently small for dates. At 36 weeks she awoke with a rush of amniotic fluid, but she did not go into labor until a week later. Her pattern was slow and intermittent, with strong, businesslike contractions for some hours followed by intervals of lower intensity and then back again. At 7 cm. she went into "back labor" with the head posterior and a nasty pain in her left sacrum and buttock, which she rubbed hard for relief. Once more KALI CARB. 200 was effective within a few minutes, the head rotating anteriorly, the cervix opening to its full extent, and the baby emerging soon after with no difficulty.

Emergencies

Taking responsibility for self-care includes being prepared to recognize genuine emergencies when no physician or midwife is on hand and to administer simple first-aid measures *en route* to the hospital. I will mention a few of the most common and important of them.

1. BLEEDING

Serious bleeding before or during the first stage of labor must be distinguished from normal "bloody show," which may also consist of quantities of bright-red blood with little or no mucus at all.

Massive bleeding has two possible causes, both life-threatening to mother and baby alike. With *placenta previa*, the placenta is abnormally attached to the lower segment below the presenting part, such that raw placental surface is exposed and may be torn as the cervix dilates. Minor or partial degrees can sometimes be detected before labor or even correct themselves as effacement pulls the placenta up out of harm's way. During labor, *placenta previa* usually presents as a sudden, massive, painless hemorrhage, which may then subside just as quickly. A presumptive diagnosis of *placenta previa* requires immediate hospitalization and preparation for transfusion and emergency Caesarean section, deferring all vaginal examinations until these latter procedures are ready to be carried out if necessary.

Abruption or premature separation of the placenta is typically accompanied by massive internal as well as external bleeding, and therefore often by significant abdominal pain with exquisite tenderness, board-like rigidity, and guarding as well. Other possible signs include high blood pressure and bleeding phenomena elsewhere, on account of rapid depletion of available clotting factors. Here too, immediate hospitalization and preparations for surgery and transfusion are mandatory.

2. PROLAPSED CORD

The appearance of the umbilical cord through the vaginal opening means that compression of the umbilical vessels and fetal asphyxiation are virtually inevitable unless the presenting part is disengaged. The attendant therefore has the tedious but important job of pushing up the presenting part well out of the pelvis and holding it there *en route* to the hospital, where Caesarean section is again the treatment of choice.

3. FETAL DISTRESS

There is no certainty or agreement about how often the fetal heart rate should be monitored during the active part of the labor, but most patients want or expect it to be done semi-routinely, perhaps every hour or so in the first stage, every half-hour in the the second, and immediately and often at the first sign of trouble.

For preventing dead or brain-damaged babies, recent studies indicate that the old-fashioned fetoscope used at intervals works just as well as electronic fetal-monitoring devices (EFM) operated continuously throughout the labor.[1] Major warning signals of acute or impending fetal distress include the passage of thick meconium through the vagina and a fetal heart rate persistently below 100 per minute.

In vertex presentations, the appearance of meconium warrants immediate delivery if the fetal heart rate is also depressed, and even meconium-stained amniotic fluid with a normal heart rate needs closer monitoring, since the baby is much more likely to need resuscitation if the birth is still a long way off. In breech presentations, passing meconium is common and need not imply fetal distress. Brief drops in the fetal heart rate to 80 or 90 per minute are common during late second-stage contractions with strenuous pushing and breath-holding, and in themselves are no cause for alarm.

4. FAILURE TO DESCEND

In a small percentage of cases, the head or presenting part fails to descend or engage below the pelvic brim despite seemingly strong and healthy contractions. If the cervix remains closed, an X-ray may help to rule out abnormalities of the bony pelvis. If dilatation is sufficient to feel the head or presenting part, other complications may need to be ruled out as well:

1. a transverse or other abnormal presentation, especially a face or brow, with an unusually large baby;
2. a large fibroid tumor interfering with descent; or
3. a bicornuate uterus or other structural abnormality making vaginal birth difficult or impossible.

Most of these cases will also require Caesarean section.

SECOND STAGE

Problems of Expulsion

I have nothing further to add to the standard techniques for managing transverse arrest, persistent occiput posterior, shoulder dystocia, and breech extraction. Probably the commonest and most important second-stage complication is simple "failure to progress," resulting in forceps extraction or Caesarean section, and traceable at least in part to two wholly arbitrary policies: 1) that women be instructed to push as soon as the cervix is fully dilated; and 2) that the baby not be allowed to remain in the birth canal for more than two hours. Devised as an administrative and legal solution to the traffic problems of a busy hospital maternity service, these bureaucratic rules ignore wide individual variations in how women actually give birth when permitted to do so in their own way.

In the first place, after hours of intense and unrelenting labor, full dilatation is often followed by a rest period of several hours, when the contractions recede and the uterus becomes more refractory to stimulation. Many patients are actually hungry or sleepy at this point, or in need of simple recreation or recharging their batteries in some fashion. Pressuring women to continue without respite makes no sense even in a hospital setting, let alone at home, where the guiding principle of the experience—and indeed, the main reason for staying there—is to give individualized attention to the needs of each mother and baby at every stage.

In the second place, many women never experience any discernible urge to push, and it only adds to their frustration and lack of confidence to expect them to summon willfully an instinctive act for which their own physical experience offers no clear or compelling directions. The perennial question, "When do I push?" is thus fairly answered with an enigmatic "You'll know," or "When you're already pushing," anticipating a time when the voluntary effort need only obey the natural process that takes over automatically without external programming. Until then, the labor may be allowed to continue as before, by simply paying attention to the breath until grunting and pushing begin to break through.

Conversely, it is always appropriate for a woman to *try* to push if she feels the urge at any stage, since it is ultimately she who must discover what her feelings mean, which ones are productive and which ones not. Unending experiments of this type are precisely how our knowledge of our bodies is acquired and imprinted for future use.

Finally, my own experience has been that babies can in fact survive quite well in the birth canal for long periods of time, provided the fetal heart rate is monitored regularly and there are no signs of distress. What should not be recommended is many hours of tedious and useless pushing in accordance with a uniform expectation of how all women are supposed to give birth. The remedies to be considered for problems of expulsion are the same as those for dysfunctional labor generally and should be given on the same indications.

Preparation for Delivery

I likewise pass over the technical details of perineal care, including such important matters as how to avoid lacerations and episiotomies. Although some midwives are particularly gifted in these matters, perineal massage with hot towels is very soothing and relaxing to most people, and preparing the labia with warm olive oil and controlling the speed and force of the baby's birth with both hands will effectively prevent many tears. Episiotomy is rarely necessary other than to expedite delivery when the infant is in obvious distress, and is the source of much needless suffering and disability afterwards.

Resuscitation and Care of the Newborn

When the baby is born, the umbilical cord may be left undisturbed until it stops pulsating and the placenta separates from the uterus, typically with a substantial gush of blood. Even then, there is no rush to cut it, since the umbilical vessels promptly close off of their own accord. On the other hand, if the cord is wound tightly around the baby's neck, it should be clamped and cut immediately, without waiting for the shoulders to be born.

Although most newborn babies begin life crying vigorously to inflate the lungs, the transition to extrauterine life need not always be so abrupt. In a sizeable minority of cases, the eyes are already open at birth, the lungs already partially inflated, and the baby appears alert, curious, and not in the least traumatized or provoked. The health status of the baby should be assessed immediately, using the Apgar method of scoring five vital functions:

1. *Heart rate:* 2 for rate over 100 per minute, 1 for below 100, 0 for no heartbeat.
2. *Respiratory effort:* 2 for vigorous (crying) or stable (resting), 1 for slow or irregular, 0 for none.
3. *Color:* 2 for pink, 1 for pink body/blue extremities, 0 for blue or white.

4. *Muscle tone:* 2 for active movement, 1 for flexion of extremities, 0 for lying limp and motionless.

5. *Reflex irritability (in response to nasal suction):* 2 for cough or sneeze, 1 for grimace, 0 for no response.

Compared to a maximum score of 10, babies scoring 7 to 10 are considered normal and require no further resuscitation; those with scores of 4 to 6 are mildly to moderately depressed and will often recover with simple suctioning or brief resuscitative efforts; and those with scores of 0 to 3 are severely depressed, at high risk of death or irreversible brain damage, and require emergency transfer to a newborn intensive-care facility.[2]

Depressed babies should be suctioned through nose and mouth using a DeLee catheter or other comparable apparatus, both to activate the breathing reflexes and to remove any meconium or other secretions obstructing the airway. Meconium in the trachea should be removed immediately by laryngeal intubation and suctioning through the endotracheal tube, before mouth-to-mouth resuscitation is attempted.

Moderately depressed babies can often be revived by stimulating the bladder meridian of acupuncture: lightly touching the cervical spine with the third finger of one hand, press down firmly with the index and fourth fingers on either side, and run them vigorously down the length of the spinal column several times, or until the baby responds.

In conjunction with these first-aid measures, homeopathic remedies can play a valuable role. For newborn babies, I prefer the tiny #10 pellets delivered from the moistened fingertip, perhaps 10 or 20 per dose, directly on the tongue. In critical situations the remedy should be repeated up to every 10 seconds and changed if there is no effect after two doses.

1. ARNICA

The remedy *par excellence* for blunt trauma to the soft tissues, ARNICA is also unsurpassed for reactivating stunned autonomic reflexes and should be considered for the baby as well as the mother after traumatic birth, especially with bruising or cephalhematoma. In such cases, ARNICA given promptly after the birth can be lifesaving. (See Chapter 5.)

> *Case 10.12.* After a long back labor and hours of pushing in the posterior position, a 23-year-old woman gave birth to her second child, a boy, who seemed a little dazed and unresponsive at first with an Apgar of 7 and a large hematoma on the forehead. After a dose of ARNICA 200 he revived in a few seconds, his bruises were no longer visible by the time I left a few hours later, and he had no further problems afterward.

2. CARBO VEGETABILIS

The leading remedy for ailments from inadequate oxygenation of the tissues, CARBO VEG. is especially useful when the baby is mildly or moderately depressed, cyanotic and slow to respond, but still capable of some unassisted respiratory effort. (See Chapter 6.)

> *Case 10.13.* After a hospital birth followed by heavy bleeding, and an abortion at 16 weeks, a woman of 34 got pregnant again and was greatly troubled by nausea that persisted well into the later months with other digestive complaints of long standing, mainly an intolerance of overeating and rich food. Although troubled in her marriage and conflicted about interrupting her career, she was determined to overcome all obstacles and did finish the pregnancy without further health problems. After an uneventful first stage, she had great difficulty pushing the baby out owing to edema of the vaginal wall and finally did so only after a midline episiotomy under local anesthesia. Her baby daughter weighed eight pounds but was moderately depressed with an Apgar of 6, feeble respiratory effort, and a heart rate of 60 per minute. Brisk suctioning and paraspinal stimulation helped somewhat, but a dose of CARBO VEG. 200 immediately elicited the loud cry we were waiting for, and she pinked up within seconds and continued to thrive after that.

Case 10.14. After four years of marriage and no birth control, a 24-year-old woman became pregnant, opting for a home birth and eating a vegetarian diet in part because of low income. Although never actually anemic, she looked sickly throughout, complained of dizziness and heartburn after meals, and often missed her prenatal appointments. The labor was easy, but the baby weighed less than six pounds and was born with a long cord wound three times around his neck and meconium-stained fluid all over his body and inside his nose and mouth. With a heart rate of 90 and an Apgar of 6, he was cyanotic, grunting for air, and generally sluggish and unresponsive. One dose of CARBO VEG. 30 roused him in a few seconds. At one minute of life he was breathing normally; within five minutes he had latched onto the breast and was nursing vigorously; and he had no further problems after that.

3. ARSENICUM ALBUM

In the absence of more distinctive indications for other remedies, ARSENICUM is the best remedy in my experience for severely depressed babies who appear lifeless with little or no color or respiratory effort and otherwise destined for intensive care in the hospital. Although infrequently cited in the literature on newborns, ARSENICUM does correspond well to ailments from auto-intoxication and complaints incident to the dying process. (See Chapter 7.)

Case 10.15. With a past history of ovarian cysts successfully treated with remedies, a woman of 31 finally conceived for the first time and remained in basically good health apart from a lingering cough that required a lot of attention. After a long, slow latent phase, she went into active labor and gave birth to a seven-pound daughter without further difficulty, but the cord was wound tight around the baby's neck and had to be clamped and cut with her shoulders and body still inside. The delivery was easy after that, but she was covered with thick meconium and did not breathe, lying motionless and unresponsive for a good 30 seconds while we suctioned and massaged her without much success. A dose of ARSENICUM ALBUM 200 brought her around in a moment. Her one-minute Apgar was 8, her five-minute was 10, and she required no further assistance after that.

Case 10.16. After a healthy first pregnancy disturbed only by a series of vaginal infections, a woman of 24 went into labor and achieved full dilatation without any trouble; but the baby, who had been in the head-down position all along, was now clearly breech. Descent and expulsion were easily accomplished, with some rotation of the legs needed to free the shoulders, but the boy, although mature and fully-formed, lay pale and motionless despite vigorous suctioning and did not breathe at all. Fortunately, the heartbeat was still strong, and he pinked up immediately after a dose of ARSENICUM ALBUM 200 and a few good cries.

Although I have not yet had enough experience with them to be sure how to recognize or use them properly, I will mention a number of other remedies that have been recommended in the literature.[3]

4. ACONITE

This remedy has been recommended for extreme cases presumably with a component of fright, with the eyes wide open and staring but the heart action very weak or imperceptible. (See Chapter 5.)

5. BELLADONNA

Perhaps more for cases with neurological involvement, BELLADONNA is recommended for babies with eyes open and staring, pupils dilated, head and body hot, and limbs motionless with twitching. (See Chapter 5.)

6. CAMPHORA

Tincture of gum or rectified spirit, *Laurus camphora*, N. O. Lauraceae, camphor.

An important remedy in the treatment of epidemic cholera and other acute illnesses with profound shock or circulatory collapse, CAMPHORA is indicated in cases of severe cyanosis with coldness of body and limbs.

7. ANTIMONIUM TARTARICUM

Trituration of potassium antimony tartrate, $2[K(SbO) C_4H_4O_6] \cdot H_2O$, tartar emetic.

Widely used in the treatment of bronchiolitis and other respiratory ailments in babies and young children, ANTIMONIUM TART. is reputed to be excellent for respiratory distress associated with fluid accumulation and rattling in the lungs, as seen in meconium aspiration, immaturity, hyaline membrane disease, and the like.

8. LAUROCERASUS

Tincture of young leaves, *Prunus laurocerasus*, N. O. Rosaceae, cherry laurel.

Comparable to CARBO VEG., CAMPHORA, and ANTIMONIUM TART., LAUROCERASUS has the indications of cyanosis with gasping for breath and coldness of the body.

9. OPIUM

Tincture of gummy exudate from unripe capsules, *Papaver somniferum*, N. O. Papaveraceae, opium poppy.

Without peer as an analgesic or narcotic, OPIUM is also used homeopathically for ailments characterized by profound stupor or coma. In the newborn, it is roughly comparable to ARSENICUM for advanced states of narcosis, when the baby is pale and unresponsive.

10. DIGITALIS

Tincture of leaves in their second year, *Digitalis purpurea*, N. O. Scrophulariaceae, foxglove.

Justly renowned and still widely used in conventional medicine as a cardiac stimulant, DIGITALIS is also used homeopathically to help revive newborn infants with respiratory distress attributable to congestive heart failure or congenital heart disease.

THIRD OR PLACENTAL STAGE

Retained Placenta

Much as after achieving full dilatation, many women cease having contractions for a short time after giving birth. Barring emergency, it is seldom necessary and may make matters worse to try to extract the placenta in the absence of any expulsive effort. With a normal amount of bleeding, it is advisable to wait for contractions to resume.

By far the best way to facilitate them is simply to give the baby to nurse as soon as possible, both to supply colostrum until the milk becomes available, and to signal the pituitary to release enough oxytocin for the final tasks of labor. If the baby is not yet able to nurse satisfactorily at this point, the spouse or other friends or loved ones may be called upon to substitute.

Separation of the placenta from the uterine wall often occurs within a few minutes after the birth, with or without contractions, and is usually announced by a significant gush of blood. In most cases descent into the vagina and expulsion are readily accomplished with the aid of a few good contractions at any time after that. Like those of earlier stages, third-stage contractions should be centered primarily in the fundus or top of the uterus, which hardens perceptibly during each one but now should also remain fairly hard in between.

Excessive third-stage bleeding due to uterine hypotonicity is usually passive and insidious and may be difficult to recognize until a great deal of blood has been lost, since even normal bleeding can elicit reflex faintness and low blood pressure not at first distinguishable from the more serious forms of shock or circulatory collapse. Placental retention may also interfere with hemostasis and thus promote bleeding. While such matters can safely be postponed until after the baby is examined and put to the breast, some care and attention should be given to recovering the placenta as soon as possible after that.

Once contractions are re-established, descent of the placenta into the vagina is readily perceptible to the patient, and it is usually a simple matter to feel or see its substantial bulk lying near the outlet. As before, it is rarely necessary or advisable to urge the woman to push without any urge to do so. If the contractions are weak, delivery may be assisted mechanically by downward compression of the fundus with one hand and lifting the low-lying placenta out of the vagina with the other.

If necessary on account of excessive bleeding, the placenta may also be removed manually using sterile precautions and perhaps sedation as well. In rare cases of pathological attachment to the uterus, surgery may be required.

Homeopathic remedies can be as helpful in the third stage of labor as before, both to stimulate more efficient contractions and to promote hemostasis after the placenta is out.

1. CAULOPHYLLUM

Whatever the condition, the indications for this remedy are always the same: uterine dysfunction with marked weakness and trembling or nervous excitement. Hypotonic uterine bleeding may also be associated at this stage. (See Chapter 3.)

2. CIMICIFUGA

As before, the characteristic indications for this remedy are dysfunctional uterine contractions with mental and/or physical fragmentation, dejection, irrational fears, alternating symptoms, choreiform movements, and the like. (See Chapter 3.)

3. PULSATILLA

Likewise prescribed on the basis of its general features, PULSATILLA fits patients with the typical vasomotor instability and improvement from open air, drinking fluids, and simple affection or loving care. (See Chapter 4.)

> *Case 10.17.* After a successful home birth and a miscarriage, a 29-year-old woman finished her third pregnancy without any health problems. The labor was

very short, and she gave birth to a son with no tears, but the placenta stubbornly refused to come out. One dose of PULSATILLA 30 enabled me to lift it out with a little fundal pressure. The bleeding was insignificant, and she had no further problems.

4. SEPIA

Although classically associated with bearing-down sensations and various general indications, SEPIA is also the remedy used most often for retained placenta when there are no guiding symptoms to suggest other remedies. (See Chapter 4.)

> *Case 10.18*. After an ectopic pregnancy, a woman of 31 was in good health for her second one except for some brown spotting in the early months that stopped after KALI CARB. and SEPIA. When her membranes ruptured, she went into labor and shortly gave birth to a son, but after separating normally the placenta would not come out. A dose of PULSATILLA 10M elicited strong contractions, but the placenta would not budge until I gave her SEPIA 10M, when it slid out easily with no resistance. She had no further problems.

Other remedies are indicated as much for associated uterine bleeding as for the retained placenta itself. (See below.)

> *Case 10.19*. Already a veteran of two home births, a woman of 26 finished her third pregnancy with only minor ailments and gave birth easily after a short labor, followed by a good deal of bleeding after the placenta separated but no contractions to speak of. After one dose of SABINA 10M, the placenta came out in a few seconds, and the bleeding slowed down to a minimum. The remainder of her course was uneventful.

Perineal Contusions and Lacerations

Although extensive second- and third-degree lacerations must of course be repaired, three homeopathic remedies may also give valuable assistance in promoting wound healing.

1. ARNICA

Unequalled for blunt trauma and bruising of the soft tissues, ARNICA can be offered with confidence if contusion of the vagina has already occurred or a large baby or difficult expulsion gives ample reason to anticipate it. (See Chapter 5.)

> *Case 10.20.* After a beautiful labor, a woman of 29 gave birth to a seven-pound baby girl with only a small first-degree tear that was not repaired. ARNICA 10M was given for extensive contusions of the vaginal floor, which healed completely in twelve hours with minimal pain or soreness.

> *Case 10.21.* In her first labor a 23-year-old woman achieved full dilatation but got stuck in the second stage, giving birth only after three hours of strenuous pushing accompanied by a good deal of bleeding and the passage of large clots. ARNICA 30 effectively minimized bruising and soreness, and postpartum bleeding was nil.

2. CALENDULA

The sovereign remedy for abrasions and small lacerations of the skin and mucous membranes, CALENDULA Ø may be applied topically to open wounds of the vagina, urethra, or perineum as an ointment or aqueous solution or added to a sitz bath. All forms of CALENDULA effectively promote healing of injured tissues and prevent infection as well. After repair of perineal lacerations or episiotomies, CALENDULA ointment may also be incorporated into the dressing with gratifying results. (See Chapter 5.)

3. STAPHYSAGRIA

Excellent for surgical wounds, STAPHYSAGRIA is the remedy of choice for minimizing pain in the incision following episiotomy or Caesarean section and for preventing the long-term discomfort and morbidity often associated with these procedures. (See Chapter 6.)

Postpartum Bleeding

Preventing and correcting excessive postpartum bleeding represent true tests of the midwife's art, requiring diligence, patience, and keen judgment. In a home setting it is particularly difficult to obtain a reliable assessment of either the rate or the total amount of blood lost, because

1. the bleeding is usually passive and thus appreciable only with the passage of time, and

2. even an average loss of 400 to 500 cc., roughly 1 pint, is sufficient to elicit reflex faintness, chills, shaking, and low blood pressure that may be virtually indistinguishable from profound shock or circulatory collapse resulting from bleeding of twice that amount or more.

Careful study of remedies can help cut through these difficulties in two ways. First, the remedy indicated by the totality of symptoms will be equally effective regardless of the extent or rapidity of the bleeding, suggesting that in most cases the distinction is purely quantitative. Second, the choice of a remedy often includes a working hypothesis about possible contributing factors such as dysfunctional labor, uterine atony, traumatic birth, retained placenta, or pre-existing bleeding tendencies, and thus suggests an appropriate strategy for management as well. In serious cases, manual or surgical removal of the placenta, blood transfusion, and other emergency measures may also be required.

1. CAULOPHYLLUM

As always, the relevant indications for this remedy include dysfunctional labor past or present with uterine atony, generalized weakness, exhaustion, and trembling or other evidence of nervous excitement. After-pains may be felt as cramps or spasms low in the pelvis or bearing-down sensations, while the fundus remains atonic and flabby and the bleeding may trickle out insidiously and be readily overlooked until quite a lot has been lost. CAULOPHYLLUM should be considered whenever the picture is dominated by excessive weakness and nervous excitability of the reproductive organs under the peak stress of labor and childbirth. (See Chapter 3.)

2. CIMICIFUGA

The classic indications for CIMICIFUGA consist of dysfunctional uterine contractions accompanied by bizarre alternations, fears or negativism, choreiform movements, or headaches, neuralgias, or joint and muscle pains. It should be considered when the freaky or random jumble of symptoms evokes a sense of mental, emotional, and physical fragmentation that will often be alarming to the patient herself as well. (See Chapter 3.)

> *Case 10.22.* After a difficult first pregnancy hampered by endless doubts and complaints, a 28-year-old woman finally went into labor. At the peak of the first stage and again in the second, her old defeatism came back but resolved each time with the help of CIMICIFUGA 200. Her nine-pound son and massive placenta were followed by a substantial amount of thin, liquid bleeding which slowed to a trickle after CHINA 200. Once her pulse and blood pressure had stabilized, I suggested CIMICIFUGA 200 four times a day, and she reported minimal bleeding and discomfort afterwards, with no further emotional difficulties of any kind.

3. PULSATILLA

Indicated as always by its general characteristics, PULSATILLA should be considered when the bleeding is accompanied by typical keynotes such as flushing or mottling, desire for cool, fresh air, and improvement from affection or reassurance. (See Chapter 4.)

4. SEPIA

Also indicated by its general symptom-picture, SEPIA will come to mind because of strong bearing-down sensations or actual prolapse, accompanied by other keynotes such as irritability with friends or loved ones, or nausea from motion or the smell or thought of food, paradoxically relieved by eating something. (See Chapter 4.)

5. ARNICA

ARNICA will often be the remedy of choice for excessive bleeding following an excessively rapid or traumatic birth, prolonged or difficult pushing, large baby, shoulder dystocia, difficult forceps extraction, or simple bruising, soreness, and depression of the normal hemostatic reflexes. (See Chapter 5.)

> *Case 10.23.* Following a successful hospital birth, a woman of 37 elected to have her next child at home and went into labor and delivered so fast that I barely made it in time. A tiny second-degree laceration was easily repaired, but she continued to bleed rather heavily. I gave ARNICA 30 every two hours for four doses and then four times daily for two days, with excellent results: the bleeding quickly subsided, and she had no further problems.

6. ACONITE

The literature recommends ACONITE for vigorous arterial bleeding associated with bounding pulse, fear of death, and other typical symptoms marked by suddenness and violence.[4] (See Chapter 5.)

7. BELLADONNA

BELLADONNA is also mentioned for bright-red bleeding so acute and forceful that the blood feels hot when it gushes out,[5] with hot, red face, dilated pupils, wild-eyed expression, or bursting headache worse from jar. (See Chapter 5.)

8. PHOSPHORUS

In patients with an underlying bleeding disorder, this remedy should be considered when other important keynotes are present, such as extreme thirst for cold drinks, fear of being alone, overactive imagination, and so forth. (See Chapter 7.)

9. IPECAC

Useful in nausea of pregnancy and other ailments accompanied by severe or constant nausea, IPECAC is also cited in the literature for vigorous, bright-red uterine bleeding after childbirth, even without nausea or other guiding symptoms.[6] (See Chapter 8.)

10. SABINA

One of the leading remedies for postpartum bleeding, SABINA is especially useful in heavily built patients with florid complexion, flushing of the face, and intolerance of heat. The bleeding is typically forcible or gushing, with bright-red blood and dark clots, and many patients complain of typical girdle-like pains from sacrum to pubis in the process of expelling them. Retained placenta or after-pains may also complicate the picture.

SABINA is also useful in late bleeding or hemorrhage a week or more after the birth and for subinvolution or bleeding that continues until the time of the six-week visit, even when there are no more distinctive indications for other remedies. (See Chapter 8.)

> *Case 10.24.* A 22-year-old woman gave birth to her first child, a six-pound baby girl, after a short, easy labor with her mother and husband both in loving attendance. The placenta came out easily even before the cord was cut and appeared grossly intact, but she bled quite heavily afterwards, and two doses of SABINA 30 were needed to stabilize her blood pressure and reduce the flow to manageable levels. When the fundus remained soft despite my efforts to massage it and her pulse rapid and thready even after CHINA 200, I emptied the uterus manually, removing several large clots and membranous fragments, and was finally able to leave her with SABINA 30 every three hours. From then on, she made a speedy recovery and had no further problems.

11. CHINA

The botanical source of quinine and the object of Hahnemann's original proving from which homeopathy was developed, CHINA was then and remains today a splendid remedy for the treatment of malaria and other intermittent fevers with chills, bone aches, dizziness, and sweating.

In homeopathy it is also invaluable for passive uterine bleeding secondary to muscular fatigue and general exhaustion with persistent oozing of dark, thin, or even watery blood. In such cases, the leading indications are much the same shock-like symptoms as would be expected from excessive blood loss: faintness, thirst, and extreme chilliness with nervous shivering and relief from warmth in any form. Other confirmatory symptoms include gassy distention of the abdomen and headache, neuralgia, or after-pains with heightened sensitivity to touch, noise, or other external stimulation.

CHINA is also unequalled as a restorative later in the postpartum period for persistent weakness or exhaustion following excessive loss of blood and more generally for ailments from loss of other body fluids as well, such as after prolonged nursing or diarrhea or gastroenteritis with dehydration. (See Chapter 8.)

> *Case 10.25.* Despite a history of chronic fatigue and considerable anxiety about her health, a 25-year-old woman remained generally healthy throughout her first pregnancy, with some help from PULSATILLA and a good deal of reassurance. After a labor that seemed in retrospect almost too easy, she gave birth to a seven-pound daughter followed by a hugely oversized placenta and large volumes of thin, dark blood that poured out of her as if from a faucet. CHINA 200 all but stopped the flow within seconds, but she needed several more doses before I dared to leave, with her blood pressure and pulse hovering around 90/60 and 120 per minute for several hours. On nothing but iron supplements for a month, she recovered quickly with no problems or sequelae, her energy returning to normal levels well before the time of her six-week visit.

> *Case 10.26.* With a history of bleeding after her first birth, a woman of 29 suffered a lot both physically and emotionally with her second pregnancy but responded well to NATRUM MUR. and other supportive measures, seeming almost radiant in the final months. The labor also went well, and the baby was fine, but the placenta separated in several jagged pieces, followed by an avalanche of dark, watery blood. Within seconds she became dizzy, faint, and cold, with a blood pressure of

60/40 and a thready pulse that was difficult to obtain. The bleeding was brought under control with PULSATILLA and other remedies, but fragments of membrane and tissue were still coming out, and it took another five hours for her vital signs and general condition to stabilize enough that I could leave. She continued to improve after that but very slowly, and when I saw her a week later she was still faint and visibly pale and exhausted whenever she stood up. CHINA 200 was wonderfully restorative, her energy quickly rebounded to normal, and there were no further complications, although she did need SILICA 200 to help with cracked nipples as well as frequent reassurance for all her customary worries.

Case 10.27. After two abortions, a 23-year-old woman got pregnant again and decided to go through with it, although still not completely "ready" to have a child. She did quite well on the whole, despite a few minor complaints that responded to the usual remedies and some third-trimester bleeding that subsided after SABINA 200. Early in labor she was hospitalized for volumes of meconium-stained fluid accompanied by late decelerations. Though she progressed rapidly and delivered a healthy baby, she bled heavily on the delivery table and signed out against medical advice the next day, with a hematocrit of 24%, after the obstetrician on call had ignored her requests and treated her abusively as well. She recovered rapidly on daily doses of CHINA 200, her hematocrit climbing to 35 within ten days without iron supplements. Although her milk supply was a little thin for the first few weeks, she nursed the baby successfully for ten months without interruption.

2. SECALE

Tincture of spurred rye, *Secale cornutum*, N. O. Gramineae, containing the fungus *Claviceps purpurea*, N. O. Fungi, ergot.

Associated since medieval times with outbreaks of poisoning characterized by gangrene and peripheral vasospasm, ergot and its derivatives ergotamine, ergonovine, and methylergonovine are still used in conventional medicine for the treatment of migraine and to promote uterine contractions and hemostasis after childbirth. Another experimental analogue, lysergic acid diethylamide or LSD, is hallucinogenic.

Ergonovine (Ergotrate) and methylergonovine (Methergine) are dangerous drugs and should never be given for retained placenta, since they produce continuous or tetanic contractions of the uterus and are likely to imprison any pieces of membrane or tissue left inside. Homeopathic SECALE is used for patients with serious bleeding, tetanic uterine contractions, and evidence of peripheral vasospasm especially in the trunk and limbs, which are typically cold to the touch yet need cold applications and cannot tolerate heat in any form.

CHAPTER 11

The Newborn Period

Once the midwife has gone and the parents are left to care for their baby, what was once a goal has become a new beginning with no end in sight. Lest the equally important subjects of childhood and child-rearing interpose themselves at this point, I have limited this concluding chapter to conditions and remedies that pertain to the first month or so of life, when the climactic events of birth are over but even more momentous adjustments must now be made on an almost daily basis.

POSTPARTUM CARE

After-Pains

Under hormonal stimulation and especially in response to nursing, the postpartum uterus continues to contract down on itself for many days, maintaining hemostasis and gradually reverting to its non-pregnant size. Typically painless, these contractions can otherwise be assessed according to the same standards as those of labor, the more painful or dysfunctional of them being likewise felt lower in the pelvis and often associated with hypotonicity and excessive bleeding as well. The appropriate homeopathic remedies and their indications are also much the same as for dysfunctional labor and postpartum bleeding. (See Chapter 10.)

1. CAULOPHYLLUM

Whatever the complaint, the total symptom-picture of this remedy includes the same basic features: uterine dysfunction (spasmodic, unstable, ineffective contractions), muscular weakness, generalized exhaustion, and nervous excitement. Often this pattern has already become evident during labor and simply continues or reappears for a time afterwards. (See Chapter 3.)

2. CIMICIFUGA

Another important remedy for after-pains, CIMICIFUGA has violent spasms or neuralgias felt low in the pelvis and typically unstable, darting about or alternating with other symptoms such as insane fears, dejection, or coarse involuntary movements in a manner indicative of physical and mental fragmentation. (See Chapter 3.)

> *Case 11.1.* A 23-year-old woman became pregnant two years after an abortion followed by excessive bleeding and a pelvic infection, an experience so unpleasant that the thought of repeating it made her violently dizzy and nauseated with guilt and self-reproach. In excellent health until the final weeks, as the birth drew near she began to complain of fatigue, restless sleep, and scary dreams in which she would be forced to endure various penitential ordeals for the baby to survive unharmed. PULSATILLA 1M was wonderfully soothing to her, and she gave birth to a fine son after a short, easy first labor with no bleeding or tears. Later that day she phoned because of severe after-pains that evoked many of the feelings she remembered since the abortion, and CIMICIFUGA 200 was splendidly effective, although it had to be repeated for several days. An episode of painful uterine bleeding and clotting one month later stopped almost immediately after the same remedy was given, and she had no further difficulties.

3. PULSATILLA

For after-pains, the general indications for this remedy are much the same as for other conditions, namely, emotional and vaso-motor instability, intolerance of warm rooms, overeating, and rich foods, and improvement from cool or fresh air, drinking fluids, and simple caring or emotional support. (See Chapter 4.)

4. SEPIA

SEPIA should be considered if the pains are felt primarily as a heaviness or bearing down as though the uterus would fall out, or are accompanied by some degree of actual prolapse or retroversion, cystocoele or rectocoele. Other typical features such as sagging of muscles and tissues generally, impatience or irritability with loved ones, and improvement from vigorous exercise or being alone will often help to differentiate the remedy. (See Chapter 4.)

5. ARNICA

ARNICA should be thought of whenever the pains follow a difficult labor or traumatic birth (Pitocin induction, precipitate delivery, hard pushing, large baby, Caesarean section) and are accompanied by bruising, soreness, or excessive bleeding into the tissues. (See Chapter 5.)

6. SABINA

Usually associated with excessive bleeding and clotting, SABINA should be considered when the patient is overheated or intolerant of warmth, and the pains girdle the pelvis and accompany the passage of large clots or placental fragments. (See Chapters 8, 10.)

7. CHINA

Also useful for after-pains with excessive bleeding, CHINA is indi-cated for many complaints attributable to dehydration from loss of blood or body fluids and associated with shock-like symptoms of prostration, chills, faintness, thirst, and hypersensitivity to touch, noise, and external stimulation generally. (See Chapter 10.)

Prolapse

Often foreshadowed by the family history, or by tendencies already evident in the past, excessive stretching or tearing of the suspensory ligaments of the pelvis during childbirth can result in actual prolapse or retroversion of the uterus. Injury or traumatism to the supporting tissues of the bladder or rectum can similarly lead to acute prolapse of the rectum through the anal opening or chronic sagging of the bladder or rectum into the vaginal vault (cystocoele, rectocoele). While surgical repair of these displacements can be very helpful when indicated, many correct themselves spontaneously or can at least be substantially relieved with homeopathic remedies if recognized and treated early enough.

1. SEPIA

The first remedy to be thought of for abnormal heaviness or dragging, pulling, or bearing-down sensations in the pelvic organs, SEPIA is unequalled in the treatment of uterine prolapse or retroversion and many other postpartum complaints as well. Other typical features like irritability with loved ones, desire to be alone, nausea better from eating something, and general improvement from physical exercise will help to confirm the selection. (See Chapter 4.)

> *Case 11.2.* After a home birth with late bleeding that stopped promptly after CAULOPHYLLUM 200, a woman of 29 became pregnant again and once more enjoyed excellent health from the beginning. Although greatly annoyed by periodontal disease, heartburn, and overheating in the final months, she responded beautifully to SULPHUR 10M, and her labor was fast and easy, as was the first. The next day she called back distraught because of "an enormous weight" that proved to be the uterus protruding out of the vagina and felt even worse when she urinated. After manual repositioning I gave her SEPIA 200, three doses in 24 hours, and by then the prolapse had corrected itself without mechanical support and did not recur. The rest of her postpartum course was uneventful.

2. ARNICA

Always to be considered after difficult or traumatic birth with bruising or soreness, ARNICA can prevent or speed recovery from the temporary bladder paralysis that may follow such an injury and would probably require catheterization if the remedy did not work. (See Chapter 5.)

3. CAUSTICUM

Tincture of impure potassium hydrate (mostly potassium hydroxide, KOH), prepared from a distilled mixture of calcium hydroxide (slaked lime, $Ca(OH)_2$) and potassium sulfate (K_2SO_4).

One of the few homeopathic remedies not found in nature, CAUSTICUM is a common laboratory reagent transformed by Hahnemann's chemical genius into an important remedy for the treatment of the chronic diseases. While its detailed pathogenesis lies well beyond the scope of this book, it deserves mention as an important remedy for Bell's palsy and other isolated paralyses of single muscles or muscle groups, including those of the larynx, throat, tongue, face, and urinary bladder. Many CAUSTICUM patients are sensitive to cold wind. For patients unable to void after giving birth, CAUSTICUM is the first remedy to be thought of if ARNICA fails or is not indicated.

4. OPIUM

One of the great medicines of human history, opium as a narcotic and analgesic is rivalled only by its own alkaloids such as morphine and codeine; semisynthetic derivatives like heroin and dilaudid; and wholly synthetic analogues like Demerol and methadone. All of these drugs are now known to act on special receptors for opiate-like "endorphins" produced in the brain itself.

Homeopathic OPIUM is useful for ailments associated with painlessness, stupor, and coma, and thus also for paralysis of the intestines or urinary bladder following Caesarean section, hysterectomy, or any other surgical procedure under general anesthesia. (See Chapter 10.)

Case 11.3. Three weeks after a seemingly normal
hospital birth in another town, a woman of 32 developed
severe abdominal pain, and a friend of hers prevailed on
me to see her at home because she was "too sick to
move." Upon entering the house I was greeted by the
stench of a massive septic infection emanating from
behind the closed door of the bedroom over thirty feet
away. With a fever of 102°F. and a pulse of 120 per
minute, the patient lay close to death, her abdomen rigid
and immobile, and her sensorium cloudy and dreamlike.
Hospitalized by ambulance, she underwent an emergency
hysterectomy that cost her both ovaries and tubes as well
as the uterus, but she did amazingly well until the third
post-operative day, when Intensive Care reported a
urinary output of only 200 cc. in the past twelve hours.
Even on massive doses of Demerol she was alert and
apprehensive when I saw her, perhaps realizing only then
how close to death she had been. I gave her OPIUM 200,
one dose, and two hours later she had diuresed 600 cc.
Her output remained normal thereafter, and she made an
excellent recovery.

5. RUTA

Most commonly used in first aid for sprains, bone bruises, and
injuries to the periosteum and other connective tissues, RUTA is
also excellent for prolapse of the rectum following childbirth,
which often corrects itself even without remedies but will do so
much more quickly with their help.

Case 11.4. After some early nausea, a woman of 26 was
disabled for much of her first pregnancy by her old back
pain, mostly a stretching or pulling sensation that was
aggravated by sitting, relieved by hot baths, and as her
labor approached was as bad as it had ever been. Her
labor was remarkably short and easy, and she gave birth
to a seven-pound son without any trouble, but by the
next day her rectum was protruding from the anal

opening by at least an inch or so. RUTA 200 was superbly effective in this most annoying situation: the prolapse corrected itself completely within a day and a half, and her back improved considerably with the help of other remedies and a series of rolfing treatments.

Phlebitis

Rarely a problem after labor, varicosities of the superficial veins tend to be aggravated by the increased blood volume and pelvic congestion of late pregnancy and to recede gradually after the birth. Inflammation of the deep veins of the thigh or calf, on the other hand, is not uncommon in the hospital, particularly after Caesarean section or in seriously ill patients, and is usually preventable by early ambulation as soon as possible after the birth.

Beginning as soreness and purplish swelling along the track of the affected veins, phlebitis may progress to swelling and pain of the whole thigh or calf with palpable or visible clots, and often fever, chills, and malaise as well. Early treatment is imperative because of the risk of serious complications, chiefly acute pulmonary embolism and chronic venous insufficiency, in which the affected leg becomes swollen, discolored, and subject to stasis ulcers and other sequelae of venous obstruction or stagnation.

1. PULSATILLA

An excellent remedy for the veins and capillaries, PULSATILLA should be considered for changeable symptoms and other typical features like flushing; sensitivity to warm rooms, unkind words, and overeating; and improvement from cool, fresh air, drinking liquids, and simple caring or emotional support. (See Chapter 4.)

2. ARNICA

This indispensable remedy can be useful preventively after difficult or traumatic births with bruising and soreness in the thighs or elsewhere. (See Chapter 5.)

3. CARBO VEGETABILIS

Another good venous remedy, CARBO VEG. represents imperfect oxygenation attributable to inadequate circulation of the blood or intestinal putrefaction from overeating or after overly rich or spoiled food. Its classic indications include indigestion with gas and venous stagnation with cyanosis, general sluggishness, and air hunger. The body and limbs are cold to the touch, but the patient is relieved by fanning or exposure to cold, fresh air. (See Chapter 6.)

4. LACHESIS

Associated with bleeding and clotting phenomena and fragility of the veins and blood vessels in general, LACHESIS is particularly indicated by predominantly left-sided complaints aggravated during or after sleep and by touch or tight clothing, and relieved by some kind of secretion, excretion, or discharge. (See Chapter 7.)

5. HAMAMELIS

Unsurpassed for simple injury or traumatism to the veins from childbirth or any other cause, HAMAMELIS is the remedy of choice when phlebitis appears imminent or threatening or there are no clear or distinctive indications for other remedies. (See Chapter 9.)

> *Case 11.5.* A 32-year-old woman finished her second pregnancy in good health after a period of depression early on that was helped a lot by NATRUM MUR. and SEPIA. The labor was more difficult than either of us expected, especially the last two hours of strenuous pushing, for which she was unprepared and out of condition. Within 48 hours she developed a fever of 101.6°F. with chills and swelling and tenderness of the left femoral vein, by then clearly visible and palpable as a thick blue cord extending halfway down her thigh. This threatening situation was promptly defused with the aid of HAMAMELIS 200, the inflammation subsiding after the first dose; within twelve hours she was fully

recovered. There were no recurrences or sequelae, and the remainder of her post-partum course was uneventful.

Postpartum Infection

Originally a disease of poor sanitation and still an important cause of maternal death in the developing countries, postpartum infection in the United States today is overwhelmingly a disease of hospitals, where the use of potent drugs and antibiotics depresses immune functions and selectively breeds highly resistant organisms. In healthy and well-nourished home birth populations, infections are quite rare if the midwife is careful not to introduce unfriendly foreign bacteria into the vaginal environment. Other risk factors include retained placental fragments, difficult or traumatic birth, poor nutrition and personal hygiene, and pre-existing chronic illness or a weakened immune system.

Often the earliest sign of infection is a change in the character of the lochia from its normally pungent odor to something more distinctly putrid or rotten, and perhaps containing slimy mucus or blood as well. Systemic symptoms like fever, chills, joint pains, and muscle aches warn of further extension into the blood and lymphatic system. The advanced picture of pelvic abscess or generalized peritonitis with board-like rigidity of the abdominal muscles and clouding of the sensorium calls for immediate hospitalization and intensive medical and surgical treatment. Especially valuable in the early stages, homeopathic remedies may also be helpful in more serious or advanced cases as a supplement to conventional treatment.

1. ARNICA

Not to be ignored in cases of difficult or traumatic birth, ARNICA is also unexcelled for ailments involving depression of the normal immune mechanisms following blunt trauma to the soft tissues. Under these circumstances, it not only promotes wound healing but can help to prevent and treat infections, abscesses, and septic states with clouded sensorium, stupor, or delirium, when the patient fails to appreciate the gravity of her illness. (See Chapter 5.)

2. CALENDULA

Applied topically for the most part and unequalled in the healing of abraded and lacerated tissues, CALENDULA also helps to prevent wound infections from an episiotomy, laceration, or surgical incision and to heal such infections once they are established, in which case it may also be given orally. (See Chapter 5.)

3. STAPHYSAGRIA

Used routinely after episiotomy and Caesarean section to minimize pain in the incision, STAPHYSAGRIA also promotes healing and helps to prevent infection following surgery of any kind. (See Chapter 6.)

4. BRYONIA

A leading remedy for appendicitis, BRYONIA is invaluable in all forms of peritoneal infection with severe pain aggravated by the least movement, low delirium or stupor, thirst, and analogous pains elsewhere in the bones, muscles, and joints. (See Chapter 6.)

> *Case 11.6.* After a successful home birth, a woman of 28 became pregnant again with a Lippes Loop still in place that I was not able to remove. Although bothered by diarrhea, leg cramps, and varicose veins for much of her pregnancy, she did improve with CALCAREA CARB. and nutritional counseling and remained generally healthy otherwise. After a short, easy labor she produced a strapping nine-pound daughter with no problems of any kind, but the IUD was still nowhere to be found. About two weeks later, after a steak dinner, she developed a burning pain in the stomach followed by weakness, muscle aches, and severe pain much lower in the abdomen. When I saw her the next day, the pain was sharply localized in the right lower quadrant over McBurney's point, felt worse from a deep breath or the slightest movement, and was accompanied by a fever of 101.2°F., chills, and a pulse of 120 per minute. The painful area was exquisitely tender, but there was no

guarding or rigidity elsewhere. After a few doses of
BRYONIA 200, this whole appendicitis-like illness
evaporated in less than 36 hours. Her IUD was later
found embedded deep within the uterine wall and had to
be removed surgically.

5. LACHESIS

In advanced infections requiring conventional treatment, the
guiding indications for LACHESIS would include hemorrhagic or
thrombotic phenomena (purpura, septic shock, DIC) and predominantly left-sided complaints, all aggravated during or after
sleep and relieved by external bleeding or discharge. (See Chapter 7.)

6. ARSENICUM ALBUM

Also a remedy for more advanced cases, ARSENICUM should be
considered for endotoxic shock or other septic states with typical keynotes such as anxious restlessness, extreme chilliness and
prostration, thirst, and burning pains paradoxically relieved by
heat. (See Chapter 7.)

7. PYROGENIUM

Tincture of purulent material from an abscess, or from meat left to
decompose in the sun, pus.

An epitome of homeopathic philosophy, PYROGENIUM is a
by-product of illness tamed by dilution and succussion into a
harmless and useful medicinal agent. Derived from ordinary pus,
PYROGENIUM is indispensable in the treatment of severe or ful-
minant infections like peritonitis, endocarditis, or septicemia,
particularly in immunocompromised patients at the mercy of their
own bacteria or fungi, when antibiotics alone may be insufficient.

Above all, PYROGENIUM is unrivalled in its ability to prevent or reverse incipient or threatening postpartum infections
associated with retained decidual or placental fragments. If the
lochia turns foul or the woman develops fever or chills a few days
after giving birth, PYROGENIUM 200 will often abort the illness
before more distinctive symptoms appear, and most patients will

recover without complications or sequelae requiring drastic conventional treatment.

In more advanced cases, its specific indications include putrid or cadaverous odors, depressed sensorium, generalized aching and soreness, and a paradoxical slowing of the pulse as the fever rises and acceleration of the pulse as the fever subsides.

Case 11.7. After an unhealthy first pregnancy complicated by malnutrition, a 24-year-old woman gave birth to an undersized baby that required CARBO VEG. 200 and some resuscitation. She also bled a fair amount afterwards. Three nights later she phoned to report fever, chills, and violent cramps in the lower abdomen extending into the thigh. On exam the temperature was 101.4°F., the pulse 132 per minute, and she had marked tenderness of the left ovary and lower abdomen generally, with some guarding and rebound. The lochia did not smell particularly bad, but she was nauseated and also unusually thirsty. My treatment consisted of PYROGENIUM 200 four times daily and a solemn promise to hospitalize her if she got any worse. She slept peacefully for the rest of the night and awoke the next morning drenched in sweat but had no fever, chills, or thirst to speak of and very little pain. By that evening the illness was over, and she nursed her baby for many months without further difficulties.

Case 11.8. A 21-year-old woman had a stormy first pregnancy full of emotional problems and a difficult labor for which both KALI CARB. and CIMICIFUGA were useful. Two weeks later she reported a shaking chill, a fever of 102°F., and much foul perspiration. Although the lochia looked and smelled unremarkable, the uterus was enlarged, boggy, and diffusely tender. After a few doses of PYROGENIUM 200, this embryonic illness disappeared as swiftly as it had begun, and by the next day she was well. At six weeks she developed acute mastitis, again with a fever of 102°F., and this time BRYONIA 30 was all she needed for a full recovery.

Depression and Emotional Problems

In the newborn period, hormonal mechanisms related to nursing and involution can easily magnify the normal stress of adjusting to the new baby, and the small nuclear family unit may also lack sufficient resources and experience to make the adjustment. Many of the same emotional issues that surfaced during the pregnancy may reappear with added poignancy after the birth, and many of the remedies and their indications are likewise identical or similar to those already described. (See Chapter 8.)

1. CIMICIFUGA

An important remedy for "postpartum blues," CIMICIFUGA should be reserved for patients with excessive moroseness or negativity, strange or irrational fears, and coarsely fragmented or alternating physical symptoms like grimacing or freaky arthritic or neuralgic pains. (See Chapter 3.)

2. PULSATILLA

Never to be overlooked for emotional complaints of pregnancy or childbirth, PULSATILLA should be considered for patients whose emotional reactions are too readily adaptable to every outside force or influence at the expense of their own inner needs. The choice of this remedy should be confirmed by the typical indications like intolerance of warm rooms, overeating or rich food, or emotional excitement and improvement from cool, fresh air, drinking fluids, and simple caring or warm emotional contact. (See Chapter 4.)

3. SEPIA

Unquestionably the leading remedy for miscellaneous postpartum complaints, SEPIA is of particular benefit to women who feel overwhelmed by the responsibilities of caring for others, insufficiently appreciated for their efforts, and involuntarily or unconsciously "turned off" to their spouses and children as a result. Typical examples might include an overly dutiful wife and mother prone to exaggerated outbursts of anger or sadness or a successful professional woman ambivalent about whether or how much to defer her own career plans. In both cases, the impression is of someone worn down, dispirited, and resentful of her obligations to her loved ones, wanting to be alone and quiet, with the usual physical symptoms like bearing-down sensations in the pelvis, a loss of muscle tone in general, and a marked improvement from vigorous exercise. (See Chapter 4.)

4. IGNATIA

This remedy is often indicated in situations colored by acute grief, sorrow, or disappointment and resulting in contradictory or anatomically "impossible" symptoms. Other signs of an overly sensitive or irritable nervous system should also be present, such as craving for or intolerance of drugs and stimulants, insomnia, or simple "nervousness." (See Chapter 6.)

> *Case 11.9.* A married woman of 19 conceived as soon as she stopped taking birth control pills, became severely nauseated, and was greatly relieved by stopping all coffee, alcohol, and tobacco, all of which she had used regularly for several years. Although still grieving after her parents' divorce four years earlier, she remained in good health throughout the pregnancy, worked right up to the end, and gave birth to an eight-pound daughter without any difficulty. At ten days of age the baby had lost a pound and a half and appeared acutely dehydrated, nursing well at first but screaming and pulling away after a few seconds, while the mother, although clearly unnerved by what was happening, ate very little and seemed almost eerily calm and impassive while she tried in vain to nurse. Fortunately the baby began to thrive on bottle feedings, which the mother accepted with the same nonchalance as before. Because of all these discrepancies I gave her a round of IGNATIA 200, and to my great amazement she regained her appetite within a week, the baby was gaining weight on her milk alone, and in the months that followed they both did well

without needing any remedies or further assistance of any kind.

5. PHOSPHORUS

This remedy should be considered for patients beset by imaginary fears for their own health or arising from empathic or even tele-pathic identification with the suffering or misfortune of others. Other typical keynotes such as bleeding phenomena, burning pains, extreme thirst for cold drinks, fear of being alone or of thunder or loud noises, or a general aggravation of all symptoms as the sun goes down will usually be present. (See Chapter 7.)

6. NATRUM MURIATICUM

Often prefigured in the pregnancy or earlier in the patient's life, NATRUM MUR. corresponds to a fixed or settled pattern of grief, sorrow, or disappointment as a permanent source of numerous physical and emotional complaints. Many of these are character-ized by excessive rigidity (arthritis, colds or allergies with nasal blockage, persistent sinus headache) and an underlying sense of resignation or futility. (See Chapter 7.)

Late Bleeding and Subinvolution

Influenced by many of the same factors as bleeding immediately after the birth, late bleeding may occur in very different patterns. In one typical scenario, instead of slowing down to a tiny amount of pinkish or blood-tinged mucus and then stopping altogether, the lochia remains bloody and heavy for weeks or intermittently relapses into episodes of frank bleeding. Hypotonicity is often a fac-tor, the uterus remaining boggy and palpably enlarged.

In other cases, after seven to fourteen days of seemingly normal flow, the patient hemorrhages without warning and may require one or more transfusions and evacuation of retained placental fragments. At about four weeks, some patients report something that resembles a light period, and it becomes clear by the follow-ing month that the normal menstrual cycle has been re-estab-lished.

The principal remedies for late bleeding and subinvolution, with their main indications, are essentially the same as for excessive bleeding immediately after the birth. (See Chapters 8 and 10.)

1. CAULOPHYLLUM
See Chapters 3 and 10.

2. CIMICIFUGA
See Chapters 3 and 10.

3. PULSATILLA
See Chapters 4 and 10.

4. SEPIA
See Chapters 4 and 10.

5. PHOSPHORUS
See Chapters 7 and 10.

6. SABINA

For subinvolution with intermittent or continuous bleeding, SABINA is often effective even in the absence of more distinctive symptoms. It has also been helpful in massive late bleeding, and in heavy bleeding associated with early resumption of the menstrual period. Its specific indications include girdle-like pains while passing clots and intolerance of heat. (See Chapters 8 and 10.)

> *Case 11.10.* A large-boned woman of 25 had had two babies weighing ten and eleven pounds respectively and had menstruated within six weeks of the births. Five weeks after the birth of her third child, who also weighed more than ten pounds, she had what she first thought was a light period, but it was followed by a second episode a week later. The physical exam was unremarkable except for a small wart on the perineum near the outer labium. After one round of SABINA 200, the bleeding stopped, she settled into her normal

menstrual cycle, and she continued to feel well and nurse successfully as she had in the past.

Case 11.11. After a successful home birth, a woman of 31 became pregnant again and had few problems other than several large, bleeding hemorrhoids and a minor recurrence of genital herpes. Pelvic examination indicated several large polyps and warty tags on the cervix and a veritable forest of thick, wavy hair that had established itself all over the pubis, groins, and inner thighs. Her labor was short and easy, like the first, but two weeks later she bled quite a lot while doing light housework and came in for treatment, recalling that she had also felt tired and discouraged since a huge nosebleed several days earlier. The bleeding stopped after a few doses of SABINA 30 and did not return. There were no further problems.

7. CHINA

Another major remedy for late bleeding, CHINA speaks more to the acute or chronic after-effects of excessive or prolonged blood loss or dehydration, especially weakness, faintness, chilliness, and marked hypersensitivity to touch, noise, cold drafts, and other environmental stimuli. (See Chapter 10.)

Case 11.12. After severe nausea in the early months, a woman of 34 remained gassy, chilly, and uncomfortable for a good part of her third pregnancy. The birth was easy enough, and she revived promptly without remedies when she bled rather heavily afterward. Ten days later she sought my help for severe dizziness whenever she stood up, pounding headaches from stooping over, and steady bleeding of thin, grayish blood. After CHINA 200 she recovered completely within a day or two and continued to do well without any need for iron supplements.

Case 11.13. Still grieving the miscarriage of her first pregnancy a decade earlier, a single woman of 33 was excited to be pregnant again and having a home birth at last. After some early nausea and a few typical fears toward the end, she went into labor and delivered beautifully with no problems or complications. Five days later she came to the office because of severe after-pains in the groin and lower back accompanied by heavier bleeding, chilliness and extreme weakness that compelled her to lie down and keep warm. Her uterus was quite flabby and tender, and every attempt to massage it made her whimper and pull away. The whole syndrome improved dramatically after a few doses of CHINA 200, and she was herself again within a few days, although her milk was never quite enough for the baby and dried up altogether after six months.

Miscellaneous Complaints

A large number of postpartum ailments need not or cannot be fitted neatly into a single diagnostic category. I have therefore included a number of miscellaneous cases to illustrate the endless variety of remedy applications and the flexible but rigorous method of selecting them.

Case 11.14. After a healthy pregnancy and an easy, uncomplicated birth, a woman of 32 came for her six-week visit with a number of minor complaints, chiefly seasonal allergies with itchy eyes, nose, and palate, marked fatigue, and impatience with her three-year-old son, who stubbornly fought having to take second place to his new baby sister. With a backache and a tipped uterus as well, she was too tired to exercise, which she knew would help her, and overly exasperated with her husband if he was more than a few minutes late coming home to spell her. Quietly, almost subliminally, a few doses of SEPIA 200 helped her to make the necessary adjustments and indirectly helped her family to do the same.

Case 11.15. Although I was never able to help her nausea very much, a 33-year-old woman enjoyed excellent health throughout the rest of the pregnancy and had her second child at home after a short labor with no tears or complications. At her six-week visit she was entirely well except for a persistent, intense, pulling pain in her tailbone when she tried to rest, during sleep, and in cold, damp weather, which forced her to squirm and fidget and change position frequently. The pain disappeared after one dose of RHUS TOX. 200 and never came back. She remained healthy and needed no further treatment.

Case 11.16. Hospitalized at 38 weeks for persistent toxemia, a woman of 24 gave birth to her first child after a successful induction, but two weeks later her blood pressure was still 150/100 with 3+ proteinuria. Otherwise she had felt very well and energetic since the birth, her chief symptom being an inordinate thirst for ice-cold drinks, amounting to ten or more big glasses of water daily, combined with an unusual chilliness in the middle of summer. On the basis of this striking pair of opposites I gave her PHOSPHORUS 200, three doses in 24 hours, and within two weeks her blood pressure and urinalysis were consistently within normal limits. Her second pregnancy a year later was wholly uneventful, with no trace of hypertension, and she gave birth at home without any difficulty.

Case 11.17. After four normal births in the hospital, a 31-year-old woman had her fifth at home without any difficulty but awoke with a headache three weeks later and a dizzy sensation that felt as if the room were swaying and made her lose her balance if she moved too quickly. Although she remembered having had a similar experience for brief moments after her last birth, this time it persisted for days and made her nauseated and apprehensive. It disappeared within minutes after a dose of COCCULUS 200 and never returned.

THE NEWBORN
Umbilical Care
If the cord stump looks infected or smells foul, it may be irrigated with aqueous CALENDULA solution and dressed with the ointment afterwards. If the baby is otherwise healthy, alert, and nursing well, these measures will almost always restore healthy granulation within a day or so.

Jaundice
Owing to immaturity of the liver, a large percentage of healthy newborns become jaundiced for a few days, usually beginning on or before the third day of life. Although this so-called "physiologic" jaundice is self-limiting and in no way injurious, the serum bilirubin often reaches 15 mg. per 100 ml., a level also seen in cases of Rh or ABO incompatibility, and must therefore be differentiated from these more serious conditions. Bruising from a difficult or traumatic birth may further intensify the jaundice or cause it to appear sooner.

In cases of Rh, ABO, or rare blood-group sensitization, affected babies may appear sickly at birth or be unable to nurse, and the jaundice is likely to appear more rapidly and, if untreated, to reach a higher peak within the first 24 to 36 hours. In suspicious cases, blood tests can easily detect blood-group antibodies and increased red-cell breakdown, and serious complications can generally be avoided with intensive light therapy and exchange transfusion if necessary.

Physiologic jaundice, on the other hand, is not dangerous and requires no treatment whatsoever unless it is persistent or severe. In such cases, frequent nursing will help flush out the bilirubin quite effectively. Weather permitting, covering the baby's eyes and exposing the skin to direct sunlight for four twenty-minute periods daily is a simple and effective alternative to ultraviolet phototherapy in the hospital. On rainy or overcast days, a blue incandescent bulb or "grow light" will serve almost as well and may be used for longer periods. Homeopathic remedies are also very helpful.

1. ACONITE

Especially for jaundice appearing rapidly, ACONITE should also be tried for hemolytic jaundice in Rh or ABO incompatibility along with conventional methods. (See Chapter 5.)

2. ARNICA

Mainly as a preventive after difficult or traumatic birth, ARNICA may also be given for physiologic jaundice complicated by bruising or hematoma formation. (See Chapter 5.)

3. NATRUM SULPHURICUM

Solution or trituration of sodium sulfate, Na_2SO_4.

An important remedy in both children and adults for asthma, allergies, and other ailments that are intensified in hot, humid weather, NATRUM SULPH. is often used empirically in the absence of more specific indications for the treatment of physiologic or hemolytic jaundice in the newborn.

ARSENICUM and THUJA are complementary.

> *Case 11.18.* After a difficult first labor that I was unable to help much with remedies, a woman of 24 made rapid progress in the hospital on Pitocin by intravenous drip, the birth following with considerable force. The baby was born in good condition with no distress and perfect Apgar scores but was already yellow after twelve hours with a bilirubin of 5 mg. per 100 ml. Since he was already nursing well and gaining weight, we were content to observe him. On the third day the bilirubin reached 14, and I gave him NATRUM SULPH. 200, three doses in 24 hours, after which the jaundice faded rapidly and the boy continued to thrive.

> *Case 11.19.* After a healthy first pregnancy and a good, strong labor, a 24-year-old woman gave birth to a six-pound girl who was slow to breathe but came around nicely with a little suctioning and CARBO VEG. 30. Her Apgar at five minutes was 9. Only slightly yellow on the

third day, she was deeply jaundiced by the fifth and remained so on the seventh. Although she had already gained five ounces over her birth weight, we gave her a round of NATRUM SULPH. 200 just in case. Her color was almost normal after 24 hours, and she continued in good health.

4. CHELIDONIUM

Tincture of whole, fresh plant at flowering, *Chelidonium maius*, N. O. Papaveraceae, greater celandine.

One of the great organ remedies, CHELIDONIUM is justly renowned for its healing power over ailments of the liver and gall bladder, including hepatitis, biliary or gallstone colic, and the typical referred pain in the region of the right shoulder or shoulder-blade. It is also an excellent remedy for all types of jaundice of the newborn in which immaturity of the liver is an important factor.

LYCOPODIUM is complementary.

Jaundice appearing after the first week of life is usually attributable to a bilirubin-like pigment present in the breast milk of some nursing mothers. Although it has been known to persist for months, this "breast-milk" jaundice is harmless and requires no treatment. Other more serious causes include various congenital anomalies of the liver and biliary tract, which require specialized diagnosis and treatment.

Hemorrhagic Disease of the Newborn

Immaturity of the liver at birth may also delay synthesis of prothrombin and other blood-clotting factors for a few days and occasionally results in transient bleeding phenomena on the fourth or fifth day. I personally have never seen more than a drop or two of blood on the cord stump or in the diaper, but with prematurity or poor nutrition the risk of serious bleeding is naturally higher.

In the hospital, an injection of Vitamin K is given routinely to all newborn babies as a preventive; it could also be given orally to the mother during labor if she wishes. But I have never found it to be necessary, as long as the baby is not being circumcised or made to undergo a number of blood tests or surgery of any kind.

Homeopathic remedies can also be of service for these bleeding phenomena, and PHOSPHORUS, with its known affinity for the liver and the bleeding mechanism, would probably be a good place to start. But in my home birth practice I have yet to see a case serious enough to warrant it. There is a lot to be said for the Biblical practice of postponing circumcision until the eighth day, when the baby is better able to handle it. An equally good case can be made for not doing the procedure at all, unless there is some compelling reason.

Conjunctivitis

Bland, yellow mucous discharges from the inside corner of the eye are common in the newborn period, usually originate from a plugged tear duct, and require no treatment other than wiping clean with a warm, damp cloth.

Still used routinely in many hospitals to prevent gonorrheal ophthalmia, silver nitrate solution is highly irritating to the eyes and often produces a nasty chemical burn or a chronic conjunctivitis that can last for months. It is also totally unnecessary, since erythromycin drops work just as well with far less irritation. In my home birth practice, I used them only if the parents insisted, or there was some other pressing reason such as an active vaginal infection or suspicious-looking discharge at the time of the birth.

Otherwise healthy newborns who develop severe or persistent conjunctivitis for no apparent reason should be treated with homeopathy or conventional means by a trained professional.

Colic and Milk Intolerance

Most commonly seen in bottle-fed babies, colic or painful intestinal cramping typically occurs within an hour after feeding and tends to subside by about three months of age. Temporary inability to digest cow's milk is also an important factor in the colic of breast-fed babies, many of whom are cured or improve dramatically within days after the mother eliminates milk and other dairy products from her diet. Others will not be benefited, while a third group tolerates cow's milk without any difficulty. A sick baby rarely becomes sensitized to its own mother's milk and may have to be fed with clear liquids or nursed for a few days by someone else.

In addition to eliminating dairy products from the mother's diet, homeopathic remedies are often wonderfully effective in the treatment of infantile colic, with none of the drowsiness, sedation, and other side effects of conventional drugs.

1. CHAMOMILLA

A leading remedy for colic or periodic irritable crying in the newborn period, CHAMOMILLA also comes closest to the experience of most colicky babies that their parents would dearly love to forget. At the center of it is simple intolerance of pain in the form of anger, outrage, or extreme irritability, which can itself aggravate and prolong other associated or pre-existing complaints.

Typically red-faced and infuriated by pain, the child needing CHAMOMILLA may kick and scream loudly or perhaps wiggle or pull away from the breast if still nursing, be comforted somewhat by being carried about or taken for a ride in the car, but resume just as forcefully when put down to sleep or rest. Often accompanied by flatulence or noisy commotion of the bowels, the stools tend to range somewhere between loose and greenish to offensive diarrhea. Yet apart from and between such episodes these babies may be perfectly healthy and happy otherwise, nursing well and gaining weight normally. (See Chapter 5.)

> *Case 11.20.* A woman of 32 had her first baby in the hospital with no difficulty, but the boy developed colic at about four weeks of age. With a history of lactose intolerance herself, she stopped eating all dairy, and the baby did improve for a short time. But a week later he had his worst attack so far and had since been prone to hours of frenzied crying after nursing in the evening. Quite happy and prosperous at other times, he would suddenly yell and scream inconsolably unless carried about by his mother, while his intestines often contributed noisy protests of their own. For some unaccountable reason, the symptoms were especially

severe in windy or stormy weather. I gave one round of
CHAMOMILLA 1M and CHAMOMILLA 30 as needed,
and within a week the episodes were much shorter and
milder, except for one that was very brief but particularly
severe, after the mother had a goodly helping of ice
cream. This attack proved to be his last. By eight weeks
he was completely free of colic and continued to thrive
and develop normally.

Case 11.21. After a classic first labor, a 29-year-old
woman gave birth at home with no complications.
Although strong and lively and gaining weight normally,
at five weeks the baby developed severe colic, kicking
and screaming with pain and trapped gas and relieved a
little by riding in the car or being walked and held firmly
against the shoulder. The stools were greenish and
watery. CHAMOMILLA 1M, three doses in 24 hours, and
CHAMOMILLA 30 as needed were dramatically
effective. By eight weeks she was essentially
asymptomatic, apart from an occasional day when only
hard pressure would relieve her and COLOCYNTHIS 30
was necessary to finish the job.

2. COLOCYNTHIS

Much as in the adult variety, colic in infants that is relieved by
COLOCYNTHIS usually presents as violent cramping that forces
the child to double over or pull the knees up and is relieved somewhat by heat but especially by hard pressure. In many cases, it
will be necessary for the parent to place the child face down across
the knees and rub or massage firmly. (See Chapter 6.)

Case 11.22. A woman of 27 had her second baby at
home after a short labor with no complications. By three
weeks of age the girl was colicky almost every evening,
when she would scream and cry, throwing arms and legs
out in all directions and loudly passing gas while
straining at stool. Although only being rubbed hard or
having a bowel movement afforded her some measure of

relief, she continued to nurse well and gain weight. After a few doses of COLOCYNTHIS 30, her complaints were gone by the time of the six-week visit and did not return.

Case 11.23. A 31-year-old woman had her first baby at home after a short labor with no complications. The boy nursed vigorously, gaining weight almost from the start, but was very colicky by six weeks, especially when the mother had milk or dairy or after a parental argument. At these times he would pull his legs up hard against his body, and the mother could relieve him only by laying him across her knees and holding or rubbing his back firmly. After giving him COLOCYNTHIS 30 as needed, she reported that the colic was essentially gone within a week or two, and that she was able to eat dairy products freely after that.

3. MAGNESIA PHOSPHORICA

With the same modalities as COLOCYNTHIS but their relative importance reversed, MAG. PHOS. is indicated for colic when the baby is relieved mostly by warm applications and only secondarily by pressure. (See Chapter 6.)

4. NUX VOMICA

Often overlooked in colic, NUX VOMICA should be considered when constipation and straining are prominent features and the symptoms are relieved dramatically after a bowel movement. For confirmation, other characteristic features such as nervous over-stimulation, wakefulness, irritability, startling, and hypersensitivity to bright light and noise should also be sought. (See Chapter 6.)

Case 11.24. After seven years of trying to get pregnant, a woman of 27 conceived and had a home birth with no trouble. Although the girl was an avid nurser, she developed severe constipation and abdominal pain in the first two weeks, often appeased somewhat by being carried about but always associated with flatulence and straining at stool. CHAMOMILLA 200 was helpful for a time, but the constipation continued to get worse, the baby grunting mightily while attempting to pass a stool and breaking into a joyful smile whenever she succeeded. The mother also reported that she startled easily from loud noises or bright light. NUX VOMICA 200 was given, and within a week the child was well.

5. STANNUM

Trituration of the metal, Sn, tin.

An excellent remedy for fatiguing coughs, STANNUM is also useful for colic and neuralgic pains that appear and disappear gradually, are relieved by hard pressure, and are accompanied by great muscular weakness and exhaustion.

PULSATILLA is complementary.

6. DIOSCOREA

Tincture of fresh root, *Dioscorea villosa*, N. O. Dioscoraceae, wild yam.

Among all the remedies useful for intestinal colic, DIOSCOREA alone is reliably effective when the pain is relieved by bending backwards or arching the back.

7. AETHUSA

Tincture of whole flowering plant, *Aethusa cynapium*, N. O. Umbelliferae, fool's parsley.

Although less often indicated in the newborn period, AETHUSA is superb when infants temporarily cannot tolerate their mothers' milk, usually in the course of an acute illness, its primary indication being projectile vomiting or diarrhea almost immediately after nursing. Often dehydrated and exhausted as well, these babies typically fall asleep soon afterwards and reawaken just as hungry as before, repeating the cycle until they are severely dehydrated and too weak to nurse. Along with a diet of clear liquids and electrolytes, given intravenously if necessary, AETHUSA can be dramatically effective in such cases.

Failure to Thrive

Although often presenting acutely and sometimes wonderfully responsive to remedies, these cases can be very complicated to unravel, and require close medical supervision as well as skillful constitutional prescribing that would take us well beyond the scope of this book. An experienced professional should be consulted.

LACTATION AND NURSING

Involution

If the woman is not nursing, or the baby dies or is given up for adoption, two remedies are well known for helping women to dry up the milk and minimize the pain and discomfort of engorgement without the risk of hormonal suppression.

1. PULSATILLA

With its special affinity for the hormonal regulation of nursing, PULSATILLA is the first remedy to think of either to dry up the milk when necessary, to increase milk production when it is deficient, or to restore it when it has been suppressed by a breast infection. When indicated by the totality of symptoms, it is also splendid for swollen and tender breasts in the non-pregnant state, especially before the menstrual period.

If the woman is not planning to nurse, PULSATILLA may be given preventively and more or less routinely at the time of the birth, without waiting for its more specific indications to develop. It may also be given later as needed for the pain and discomfort of engorgement and letdown. (See Chapter 4.)

> Case 11.25. A single woman of 25 became pregnant and decided to put the baby up for adoption. The pregnancy and birth were both healthy and trouble-free, but even with a hormone injection she remained painfully engorged on the fifth postpartum day. After a few doses of PULSATILLA 30 the pain and swelling had largely subsided by the following morning, eliminating the need for more hormones or strapping.

2. LAC CANINUM

Tincture of bitches' milk, *Canis familiaris*, N. O. Carnivora, dog's milk.

Widely used for female complaints in ancient times, LAC CANINUM is used homeopathically for headaches, throat infections, breast and ovarian complaints, and other symptoms that involve both the right and left sides in alternation, proceeding back and forth between one and the other. Vertigo with strange "floating" sensations is another notable feature.

When PULSATILLA has been tried without success, LAC CANINUM is similarly useful in preventing or minimizing the pain of engorgement and may also be given semi-routinely without waiting for its more specific indications. It is equally valuable for augmenting or restoring the milk.

Cracked and Sore Nipples

Unequalled in its healing power over simple cuts and abrasions, CALENDULA preparations should be included in routine breast care and hygiene before and after the birth to help condition and toughen the nipples and areolae in preparation for nursing. Along with good nutrition, massaging the nipples regularly with CALENDULA ointment will significantly reduce the incidence and severity of cracks and soreness throughout the nursing period and thus enhance the nursing experience as a whole.

When cracks and soreness do develop, three other remedies may be considered for internal use.

1. CASTOR EQUI

Trituration of scales from the rudimentary thumbnail of the horse, *Equus caballus*, N. O. Perissodactyla.

Another remedy of ancient pedigree, CASTOR EQUI has been used for brittle nails but is said by many to be virtually specific for the cracked and sore nipples of nursing women, with a reputation for healing even advanced or "hopeless" cases. Unfortunately, having learned of it only recently, I cannot yet report on it from my own experience.

2. HEPAR SULPHURIS

Trituration of *hepar sulphuris calcareum*, an impure calcium sulfide obtained by combustion of oyster shells (mostly $CaCo_3$) with brimstone or flowers of sulphur (S), "liver" of sulphur.

A valuable remedy for boils, abscesses, impetigo, and other purulent bacterial or fungal infections, HEPAR SULPH. is useful in cracked, sore, painful nipples overgrown with Staphylococci, Streptococci, or other pus-forming organisms commonly found in the skin. In more advanced cases, its characteristic indications include irritability, chilliness, marked sensitivity to cold winds or drafts, improvement from heat or warmth in any form, and a purulent discharge or exudate often smelling like old cheese.

3. SILICA

Trituration of silicon dioxide or flintstone, SiO_2, silica.

An important constituent of the earth's crust and capable of deep, slow "constitutional" action, SILICA is especially useful in promoting the extrusion of foreign bodies and the healing of fissures, abscesses, ulcers, granulomas, fistulas, and other forms of chronic suppuration. With its cystic glands and elaborate duct system, in which unused or soured milk readily attracts needy bacteria, the lactating breast can be an excellent laboratory for the slow ulcerative and suppurative processes that call for SILICA.

In the early weeks of nursing, if the nipples are very sore and tend to crack easily, SILICA 6C may be given four times daily as needed to toughen them. When indicated, it is also an excellent remedy for the deeper cracks, lumps, and abscesses that can develop later. While its detailed chronic symptom-picture would far exceed the scope of this book, SILICA can be prescribed with confidence for unforgettably sharp, splinter-like pains in the nipple when the child nurses that often extend through the breast to the shoulder. In general it is a chilly remedy, and patients needing it are likely to be adversely affected by cold in any form.

> *Case 11.26.* After three miscarriages, a 36-year-old woman had her second child at home, worrying us a bit with a slow labor and some meconium-stained fluid, but

with normal fetal heart tones throughout. At her one-week visit she complained of sharp, needle-like pains in her right nipple when the baby started to nurse that she felt all the way through to the shoulder. Although they tended to lessen somewhat as the feeding continued, they were so intense that she had to clench her teeth or pull away and dreaded the sound of her own child each time he cried out for her. The breast nevertheless yielded plenty of milk with no lumps or fissures, and the nipple also looked normal except for a tiny spot of grayish matter covering the opening that neither of us could figure out how to remove. I gave her a round of SILICA 200 followed by SILICA 6C as needed. About a week later she reported that the pain, which had lessened for the first few days, became intolerable again during a feeding but ended abruptly when the nipple discharged a ribbon of caseous material smelling like old ear wax. The nursing was painless and trouble-free after that, and she remained in good health otherwise.

PULSATILLA is complementary.

Breast Infections

When one or more milk ducts are blocked by dried milk, the lactating breast can become vulnerable to colonization and super-infection by pus-forming organisms from the skin. The broad term "breast infection" covers a whole spectrum of clinical responses ranging from acute mastitis with high fever to more localized and chronic or relapsing phenomena such as abscesses, lumps, and fissures.

These events are best prevented and minimized by good nutrition to boost the immune system and maintain the normal skin flora in a healthy balance. A second precaution is to encourage the baby to empty both breasts at every feeding, not allowing unused milk to accumulate, sour, and harden in the duct system, which once plugged becomes a nutritious culture medium for any microorganisms that may be nearby.

Emptying the breasts also brings smiles of contentment, promotes healthy sleep, and provides the crucial stimulus for further milk production and thus for optimal growth and development as well. If necessary, a good hand-held pump can be used to extract any surplus milk, which can then be stored for future use. If either breast does become infected, hot towels may be used liberally to dissolve milk concretions and unplug any blocked or clogged ducts.

Homeopathic remedies are useful at any stage, both for treatment of acute mastitis, breast abscess, and their chronic sequelae, and also preventively, when these complications seem imminent or threatening.

1. BELLADONNA

A leading remedy for acute mastitis, BELLADONNA is especially suitable when a nursing mother suddenly develops high fever with violent throbbing or bursting pains in the breast and other signs of acute inflammation. The affected area of the breast is acutely swollen, bright-red or even shiny in appearance, and exquisitely tender and sensitive to the slightest jar, such as someone sitting down next to her on the bed. A throbbing or bursting headache, wild-eyed expression, extreme sensitivity to light and noise, and other typical features may also be present. (See Chapter 5.)

> *Case 11.27.* A 24-year-old woman had her second baby at her home in the country with no trouble. Nine days after the birth, the baby seemed much less eager to nurse, and by evening her breasts were already painfully engorged and she herself felt chilly and weak. The following afternoon she developed a fever of 103.2°F. with soreness of the left breast, a headache that throbbed with the slightest movement, and a grumpy, irritable mood. BRYONIA 30 four times daily was very effective, and she was back to normal in a few days; but four weeks later the whole thing happened again, this time in the right breast, with a fever of 103°F., a pain extending into the armpit, and a severe, pounding headache. The breast

hurt especially from bumping, touching, or lying on it, and her face was very red and swollen. This time BELLADONNA 30 was given, and within 36 hours the illness was gone without a trace and never came back. Afterwards she recalled that the baby had slept eight hours straight the night before her relapse and that she had been painfully engorged by morning.

Case 11.28. A woman of 25 had her second child at home after a surprisingly difficult labor, but everything went well until four months later, when she developed a fever of 104°F. and her left breast hurt as if it had been "hit with a baseball bat" whenever she tried to move her arm or roll over. Originating in the lower half of the breast, the pain was worse from the least movement of any kind and made her want to be left alone. BRYONIA 30 was of no value. By the next day she had a pounding headache, and for the baby even to touch the breast made her "crazy." BELLADONNA 30 was substituted at this point, there was no sign of infection by the next morning, and she remained in good health for the rest of the nursing period.

2. BRYONIA

The other great remedy for acute mastitis, BRYONIA is especially suitable when the illness develops more slowly and, in spite of its soreness, the patient may lie on the painful side to shield the breast from the smallest movement. Other typical keynotes such as extreme thirst, gruff or irritable mood, dazed sensorium, and aversion to stimulation of any kind are also likely to be present. (See Chapter 6.)

Case 11.29. After a difficult first pregnancy, a 21-year-old woman had a strong labor and a successful home birth with no complications except a fever and chills ten days later that subsided almost immediately after PYROGENIUM 200. All went well until just after her six-week visit, when her right breast became very sore and tender to the touch and she developed an unusual thirst and a fever that went up slowly during the day and reached 102⁰F. by evening. Because her breast hurt most with every step and from the slightest movement, she was forced to wear a tight bra for support and to hold herself rigidly in place. After a few doses of BRYONIA 30, her illness gradually subsided over the next 36 hours and never came back.

3. PHYTOLACCA

Tincture of ripe berries, *Phytolacca decandra*, N. O. Phytolaccaceae, poke root.

Widely praised in the herbal literature for the treatment of breast cancer, PHYTOLACCA is used in homeopathy for many ailments of the female breast and for tumors, abscesses, and inflammations of other lymphatic and glandular structures as well, particularly the throat and tonsils. An extract of the berries has also been used to accelerate fat metabolism and the breakdown of fatty tissue in selected cases of obesity and compulsive eating.

In my experience, at least three-fourths of my acute mastitis patients with high fever benefited substantially from either BELLADONNA or BRYONIA or both, and almost that many recovered completely without requiring other remedies. PHYTOLACCA has no peer in healing the assorted lumps, pains, and congestions that can easily lead to acute infection if not corrected, or are left over after the acute remedies have done their work.

The breast that needs PHYTOLACCA feels lumpy, hard, and tender in spots, and its pains frequently change location or wander to other areas of the chest or more distant parts of the body. In acute infections and abscesses, it is apt to be useful after BELLADONNA and BRYONIA have worked or failed to work, or before the symptoms are sufficiently intense or distinctive to indicate them.

> *Case 11.30.* With a history of recurrent mastitis after each one of her previous births, a woman of 33 had her fifth child at home after a short labor with no problems

268

of any kind. In less than three weeks she had a fever of 102°F., pain in the left breast from the least movement, and reduction in the milk supply on that side. The infection subsided quickly on BRYONIA 30, but her milk production continued to dwindle and was not fully re-established until PULSATILLA 30 was given four times daily for a whole week. Although her breasts continued to feel lumpy and sore thereafter, as they had throughout her long nursing career, she neglected to come back until her next acute episode almost a year later, this time with a raging fever, a hard, red lump in the left breast after a day in the hot sun, and the sensation that her breast was "burning up." Within hours after BELLADONNA 30, her fever rose to 105.6°F. and then plummeted sharply as she awoke from an out-of-body experience, but she continued to have a low fever with much sweating and a big lump that was sore to the touch and reminded her of many others she had endured in the past. At this point I gave her PHYTOLACCA 30, and the lump gradually became smaller and finally disappeared in four days, after which she was able to continue nursing without any further problems.

Case 11.31. After unsuccessful attempts to abort using pennyroyal and other herbs, a woman of 28 decided to go through with the pregnancy, her first, and eventually won over her husband as well. Apart from a number of minor complaints and the spiritual conflicts that gave her no peace, her most immediate problem was a hematocrit that went down to 31.5 in the last month and some fanatical dietary notions that made it next to impossible to reason with her. She nevertheless had a lovely home birth, and the nursing also seemed to be going well until the six-week visit, when she complained of several tender lumps in her left breast, which was also smaller and gave less milk than the right. PHYTOLACCA 30 was given, and within a month or so the lumps were gone and the left breast was full of milk and producing normally, although it had always been and remained the smaller of the two.

4. SILICA

In addition to its many uses for sore or cracked nipples, SILICA when indicated can be a valuable remedy for promoting healing of old lumps, abscesses, or draining sinuses left over from chronic or recurrent mastitis that never fully resolved. In such cases, other typical keynotes such as caseous discharges and extreme chilliness or sensitivity to cold air and drafts will ordinarily be present.

> *Case 11.32.* Late in her second pregnancy a 33-year-old woman consulted me for painful lumps in the right breast. PHYTOLACCA 30 was helpful temporarily, but by 33 weeks both breasts were huge and pendulous and the right one was a mass of hard, tender nodules, some of which had opened and were discharging fluid that looked like cream of tomato soup. She nevertheless had a successful home birth and began to nurse despite the dire warnings of two specialists that these galactocoeles would persist and become chronically infected until she weaned the baby. At this point the drainage was either yellow or milky, and she complained of frequent, sharp, needle-like pains here and there. A number of older lesions had also developed indurated areas resembling scar tissue. After two rounds of SILICA 30 a week apart, the cysts became smaller and less painful and finally stopped draining, and she was able to continue nursing until she conceived again a year later.

NOTES

INTRODUCTION

1. Cf. Brackbill, Y., *et al.*, *Medication in Maternity*, International Academy for Research in Learning Disabilities, University of Michigan, Ann Arbor, 1989, pp. 43–129.
2. Dorfman, P., *et al.*, "Preparation for Childbirth by Homeopathy," *Cahiers de Biothérapie* 94: 77–81, April 1987.

CHAPTER 1

1. The Homeopathic Pharmacopoeia of the United States (HPUS) was recognized by Congress in the Food, Drug, and Cosmetic Acts of 1938 and 1956, and is supervised by the U.S. Food and Drug Administration (FDA).
2. Cf. Hahnemann, S., *The Organon of Medicine*, Fifth Ed., with additions from the Sixth, trans. W. Boericke and E. Dudgeon, Roy, Calcutta, 1961, aphorisms 53–70.
3. The term "homeopathy" is derived from the Greek roots ομοιos or *omoios*, meaning "similar" (as in "homeostasis," the biological process whereby living organisms maintain a more or less constant internal environment), and πάøos or *pathos*, meaning "suffering" or simply "feeling" (as in "sympathy," "antipathy," "pathology," or indeed "pathos" itself).
4. Cf. Moskowitz, R., "Homeopathic Reasoning," *Homeotherapy* 6: 135–142, September 1980, reprinted by the National Center for Homeopathy, Alexandria, VA.
5. Cf. Whitmont, E. C., *Psyche and Substance*, North Atlantic Books, Berkeley, 1991, pp. 3–79.
6. Cf. Hahnemann, *op. cit.*, aphorisms 266–271, with footnotes.

7. Cf. Boiron, J., "Studies of the Physical Structure of Homeo-
pathic Dilutions Utilizing the Raman Laser Effect," *Proceed-
ings*, 31st Congress of the International Homeopathic Medical
League, Athens, 1976, pp. 459–474; Noiret, R., "Activity of
Several Homeopathic Dilutions of $CuSO_4$ in Different Micro-
bial Species," *ibid.*, pp. 137–147; and Resch, G., "Physical
Chemistry of Highly Attenuated Remedies," *Proceedings*, 42nd
Congress of the International Homeopathic Medical League,
Washington, 1987, pp. 300–304.

8. Cf. Moskowitz, R., "Some Thoughts on the Malpractice Crisis,"
British Homeopathic Journal 77: 18–22, January 1988.

9. Hering, C., "Hahnemann's Three Rules Concerning the Rank
of Symptoms," *Hahnemannian Monthly* 1: 5–12, 1865, and *Ana-
lytical Therapeutics*, Boericke and Tafel, Philadelphia, 1875, p. 24.

CHAPTER 2

1. The Homeopathic Pharmacopoeia of the United States
(HPUS), Eighth Edition, has now been superseded by a number of additions and deletions made since its publication in
1980, and the Ninth Edition has not yet been completed. The
new information has been published *seriatim* in the form of
detailed monographs written by the Homeopathic Pharmacopoeia Revision Service (HPRS).

2. In the Sixth Edition of his *Organon of Medicine*, Hahnemann
also introduced the so-called "50-millesimal" scale, based on serial dilutions of 1:50,000 each. Although these "LM" potencies are highly regarded by many, the method of preparing and
using them is somewhat cumbersome, and I am not yet sufficiently conversant with it to discuss it here.

3. Even patients who cannot tolerate lactose, sugar, or alcohol
in quantity can usually take remedies containing minute
amounts of these substances without difficulty.

4. Cf. Kent, J. T., *Repertory of the Homeopathic Materia Medica*,
Final Edition, Ehrhart & Karl, Chicago, 1946, the text most
commonly used by prescribers in this country.

5. For a fuller account of reactions to the remedy, see Kent, J. T., *Lectures on Homeopathic Philosophy*, Ehrhart & Karl, Chicago, 1954, pp. 250–284, and Vithoulkas, G., *The Science of Homeopathy*, Grove Press, New York, 1980, pp. 227–232 and 295–322.

CHAPTER 3

1. Cf. Hering, C., *The Guiding Symptoms of Our Materia Medica*, 10 vols., Hering Estate, Philadelphia, 1891.

2. Cf. Clarke, J. H., *Dictionary of Practical Materia Medica*, 3 vols., Health Science Press, Rustington, UK, 1962.

3. Cf. Dorfman, *op. cit.*, pp. 77–81.

4. Unpublished letter to the author.

CHAPTER 4

1. For the "homeopathic aggravation," cf. *supra*, Chapter 2, p. 20.

CHAPTER 7

1. Cf. Hering, C., "The Pathogenetic Power of the Snake Venom [*Lachesis muta muta*] to Provoke Disease," transl. J. Jaffe, The Homoeopath 12: 155–158, March 1992; and Knerr, C., Life of Hering, Magee, Philadelphia, 1940, p. 197. The first proving of LACHESIS was begun on July 28, 1828, and Hering died on July 23, 1880.

CHAPTER 8

1. Cf. Stewart, F., *et al.*, *Understanding Your Body*, Bantam, New York, 1987, p. 191.

2. Cf. Lust, J., *The Herb Book*, Bantam, New York, 1974, pp. 304, 376.

3. Just as the typical nausea and vomiting of pregnancy probably signifies only that these normal adaptive processes are under way, their disappearance in timely fashion implies a favorable prognosis for the rest of the pregnancy (and beyond), while pernicious vomiting extending into the later months can warn

of more serious congenital or other developmental problems at the placental level.

4. Cf., for example, *Composition and Facts about Foods*, Health Research, Mokelumne Hill, CA, 1971. Although less well known and harder to find than many others, this wonderful reference work lists each nutrient separately, enabling the reader to see at a glance how best to obtain it.

5. Brewer, G. S., with Brewer, T., *What Every Pregnant Woman Should Know*, Penguin, New York, 1979, pp. 34–75.

6. Cf. *supra*, Chapter 1, pp. 1–2.

7. Cf. *Composition and Facts about Foods*, pp. 36–37.

8. Cf. *ibid.*, p. 76.

9. Cf. *ibid.*, pp. 28–29.

10. Cf. *ibid.*, pp. 28–29.

11. Cf. *ibid.*, pp. 42.

12. Cf. Kervran, L., *Biological Transmutations*, trans. M. Abehsera, Swan House, Binghamton, N. Y., 1972, pp. 1–12, 44–47, 93–101, and 135–144.

CHAPTER 9

1. Hahnemann's monumental work, *The Chronic Diseases*, first published in 1828, occupied him for the last twenty-five years of his life. Although still controversial and by no means universally accepted even among practicing homeopaths, it is a serious attempt to classify and explain the chronic diseases of mankind. Corresponding to the remedies SULPHUR, THUJA, and MERCURIUS, his three main types represent broad pathological "styles" characterized by signs and symptoms of deficiency, excess or proliferation, and ulceration or destruction, respectively.

2. Brewer and Brewer, *op. cit.*, pp. 34–75.

CHAPTER 10

1. Cf. Leveno, K., *et al.*, "A Prospective Comparison of Selective and Universal Electronic Fetal Monitoring in 34,995 Pregnancies," *New England Journal of Medicine* 315: 615, September 4, 1986; King, D., *Boston Globe*, March 1, 1990, p. 1; and *Family Practice News*, September 15, 1991, p. 32.

2. Oxorn, H., *Human Labor and Birth*, 4th Ed., Appleton-Century-Crofts, New York, 1980, p. 691.

3. Cf. Farrington, H., "Homeopathy in the Newborn Infant," *Journal of the American Institute of Homeopathy*, 48: 145–148, May 1955.

4. Cf. Guernsey, H. N., *Obstetrics*, 3rd Ed., Hahnemann, Philadelphia, 1891, p. 406.

5. Cf. Yingling, W. A., "Some Obstetrical Thoughts," *Homeopathic Recorder* 45: 584, August 1930.

6. Cf. *ibid.*, pp. 583–584.

APPENDIX I

Suggestions for Further Reading

Many of the old textbooks have been reprinted. Those in print are available from Homeopathic Educational Services, 2124 Kittredge Street, Berkeley, CA 94704, The Minimum Price Homeopathic Books, Blaine, WA 98230, and other distributors. Old periodicals are much harder to obtain and often have to be photocopied from homeopathic collections such as those housed in the National Center for Homeopathy, Alexandria, VA; the National Library of Medicine, Bethesda, MD; the John Bastyr College of Naturopathic Medicine, Seattle, WA; the National College of Naturopathic Medicine, Portland, OR; or Homeopathic Resources and Services, Old Chatham, NY.

1. *History and Philosophy*

Coulter, H., *Divided Legacy: Science and Ethics in American Medicine*, 1800–1914, North Atlantic Books, Berkeley, 1975.

Haehl, R., *Samuel Hahnemann: His Life and Work*, 2 vols., trans. M. Wheeler and W. Grundy, Jain, New Delhi, 1971.

Hahnemann, S., *The Organon of Medicine*, 5th Ed., with Additions from the 6th, trans. W. Boericke and E. Dudgeon, Roy, Calcutta, 1961.

Kent, J. T., *Principles of Homeopathic Philosophy*, Boericke & Tafel, Philadelphia, 1954, reprinted North Atlantic Books, Berkeley, 1979.

Moskowitz, R., "Homeopathic Reasoning," *Homeotherapy* 6: 135–142, September 1980, reprinted by the National Center for Homeopathy, Alexandria, VA.

Ullman, D., *Discovering Homeopathy: Medicine for the Twenty-First Century*, North Atlantic Books, Berkeley, 1991.

Vithoulkas, G., *Homeopathy: Medicine for the New Man*, Arco, New York, 1972, paper.

Vithoulkas, G., *The Science of Homeopathy: A Modern Textbook*, Grove Press, New York, 1980, paper.

Whitmont, E. C., *Psyche and Substance*, North Atlantic Books, Berkeley, 1991, paper.

2. Methodology

Roberts, H. A., *Principles and Art of Cure by Homeopathy*, Health Science Press, Rustington, UK, 1942.

Ullman, D., and Cummings, D., *Everybody's Guide to Homeopathic Medicines*, Jeremy Tarcher, Los Angeles, revised 1991.

Ullman, D., *Homeopathic Medicine for Children and Infants*, Jeremy Tarcher, Los Angeles, 1992.

Vithoulkas, *The Science of Homeopathy*, op. cit.

Wright-Hubbard, E., "A Brief Study Course in Homeopathy," in *Homeopathy as Art and Science*, ed. M. Panos and D. Desrosiers, American Institute of Homeopathy, Beaconsfield, UK, 1990, pp. 265–340.

3. Materia Medica

Barthel, H., and Klunker, W., ed., *Synthetic Repertory*, 2nd Ed., 3 vols., Haug, Stuttgart, 1983.

Boericke, W., *Materia Medica with Repertory*, 10th Ed., Boericke & Tafel, Philadelphia, 1991.

Clarke, J. H., *Dictionary of Practical Materia Medica*, 3 vols., Health Science Press, Rustington, UK, 1962.

Coulter, C. R., *Portraits of Homeopathic Medicines: Pscyhophysical Analyses of Selected Constitutional Types*, 2 vols., North Atlantic Books, Berkeley, 1986, 1988.

Hering, C., *Guiding Symptoms*, 10 vols., Hering Estate, Philadelphia, 1891.

Kent, J. T., *Lectures on Homeopathic Materia Medica*, 4th Ed., Boericke & Tafel, Philadelphia, 1956.

Kent, J. T., *Repertory of the Homeopathic Materia Medica*, Final Edition, Ehrhart & Karl, Chicago, 1946.

Künzli, J., ed., *Repertorium Generale*, Barthel & Barthel, Berg, Germany, 1987.

Nash, *Leaders in Homeopathic Therapeutics*, Boericke and Tafel, Philadelphia, 1901.

Tyler, M., *Homeopathic Drug Pictures*, Health Science Press, Rustington, UK, 1970.

Warkentin, D., *MacRepertory* software, Kent Homeopathic Associates, San Anselmo, CA, 1992.

Whitmont, *op. cit.*

4. Pregnancy and Childbirth

Allen, H. C., "Our Hemorrhagic Friends," International Hahnemannian Association (I. H. A.) *Transactions*, 1895, pp. 290–301.

Baylies, B. LeB., "Jottings of Cases," I. H. A. *Transactions*, 1888, pp. 342–359.

Baylies, B. LeB., "PULSATILLA in Malposition of the Fetus," I. H. A. *Transactions*, 1890, pp. 133–146.

Blackmore, R., "Homeopathy in the Maternity Room," I. H. A. *Transactions*, 1909, pp. 177–186.

Close, S., "Advantages of Constitutional Treatment Preceding Conception," I. H. A. *Transactions*, 1911, pp. 277–289.

Custis, J. B. G., "The Hahnemannian Obstetrician," I. H. A. *Transactions*, 1890, pp. 107–117.

Faris, R. S., "The Use of Homeopathy in Obstetrics," *Homeopathic Recorder*, 61: 79–85, September 1945.

Farrington, H., "Homeopathy in the Newborn Infant," *Journal of the American Institute of Homeopathy* (AIH), 48: 145–148, May 1955.

Green, J. M., "The Homeopathic Remedy for the Parturient

Woman and Young Infant," I. H. A. *Transactions*, 1924, pp. 126–134.

Green, J. M., "The Sphere of the Remedy in Obstetrics," I. H. A. *Transactions*, 1916, pp. 242–247.

Guernsey, H. N., *Obstetrics*, Hahnemann, Philadelphia, 1891.

Hawkes, W., "Some Thoughts and Recollections on Obstetrics," I. H. A. *Transactions*, 1915, pp. 430–440.

Hayes, R. E. S., "The Psyche and Science," I. H. A. *Transactions* 1925, pp. 287–298.

Houghton, H. L., "The Third Stage of Labor," I. H. A. *Transactions*, 1907, pp. 224–227.

Krichbaum, J., "Homeopathic Aids in Labor," *Homeopathic Recorder* 45: 805–808, November 1930.

McLaren, D. C., "Pregnancy and Parturition: A Few Valuable Remedies," I. H. A. *Transactions*, 1886, pp. 186–90.

McLaren, K., "Tedious First Stage of Labor," *Homeopathic Recorder* 56: 219–223, May 1941.

Neiswander, H. A., "Complaints of Pregnancy," *Homeopathic Recorder* 65: 271–274, April 1950.

Pulford, A., "The Parturient Woman," *Homeopathic Recorder* 58: 493–497, April 1943.

Putnam, A. C., "Homeopathic Obstetric Forceps," I. H. A. *Transactions*, 1913, pp. 298–301.

Rabe, R., "Medication during Parturition," I. H. A. *Transactions* 1911, pp. 289–293.

Roberts, T., "Some Homeopathic Remedies for Puerperal Infection," I. H. A. *Transactions*, 1908, pp. 262–268.

Schmitt, J., "High Potencies in Parturition," I. H. A. *Transactions*, 1884–1885, pp. 142–152.

Schwartz, F. A., "Homeopathic Remedies in Obstetrics," *Homeopathic Recorder* 55: 20–25, May 1940.

Schwartz, F. A., "Homeopathic Remedies in Obstetrical Complications," *Homeopathic Recorder* 59: 19–22, July 1943.

Sherbino, G., "Obstetrical Cases," I. H. A. *Transactions*, 1890, pp. 146–150.

Stevens, G., "Homeopathic Treatment during Lactation," I. H. A. *Transactions*, 1911, pp. 294–299.

Sutherland, A., "Hyperemesis Gravidarum," *Homeopathic Recorder* 53: 3–9, July 1938.

Villers, A., "On Habitual Miscarriage," I. H. A. *Transactions*, 1895, pp. 264–275.

Winans, T., "How the Similar Remedy Aided Me in Getting an Obstetrical Practice," I. H. A. *Transactions*, 1917, pp. 518–524.

Winans, T., "Vomiting in Pregnancy," I. H. A. *Transactions*, 1914, pp. 361–369.

Woodbury, B., "Some Problems of the Obstetrician," I. H. A. *Transactions*, 1918, pp. 248–262.

Woodruff, M., "Some Obstetrical Experiences of One of the Veterans," I. H. A. *Transactions*, 1909, pp. 164–168.

Yingling, *Accoucheur's Emergency Manual*, Boericke & Tafel, Phila., 1894; reprinted Sett Dey, Calcutta, 1968.

Yingling, W. A., "Retained Placenta," I. H. A. *Transactions*, 1901, pp. 301–309.

Yingling, W. A., "Homeopathic Treatment during Pregnancy," I. H. A. *Transactions*, 1911, pp. 300–305.

Yingling, W. A., "Some Obstetrical Thoughts," *Homeopathic Recorder* 45: 580–586, August 1930.

INDEX

About the Author

Richard Moskowitz, M.D., completed his undergraduate degree at Harvard and his medical education at New York University. A past President of the National Center for Homeopathy and a regular member of their teaching faculty, Dr. Moskowitz has contributed more than forty articles and interviews to the *Journal of the AMA*, *Mothering*, *Natural Health*, *Chrysalis*, and various homeopathic journals in the U. S. and abroad. With a homeopathic experience spanning eighteen years and over eight hundred pregnancies, he is currently engaged in a homeopathic family practice in Watertown, Massachusetts.